OUR LONG MIDNIGHT

Reflections of a Physician on Life and Faith During a Global Pandemic

By Dr. Jean Chamberlain-Froese, CM, MD, FRCSC

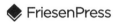
FriesenPress

One Printers Way
Altona, MB R0G 0B0
Canada

www.friesenpress.com

Copyright © 2022 by Dr Jean Chamberlain-Froese
First Edition — 2022

All rights reserved.

No part of this publication may be reproduced in any form, or by any means, electronic or mechanical, including photocopying, recording, or any information browsing, storage, or retrieval system, without permission in writing from FriesenPress.

Unless otherwise credited, all photographs are by Jean Chamberlain-Froese or Thomas Froese.

Scripture taken from the HOLY BIBLE, NEW INTERNATIONAL VERSION®. Copyright © 1984 International Bible Society. Used by permission of Zondervan. All rights reserved.

ISBN
978-1-03-911552-1 (Hardcover)
978-1-03-911551-4 (Paperback)
978-1-03-911553-8 (eBook)

1. RELIGION, DEVOTIONAL

Distributed to the trade by The Ingram Book Company

Table of Contents

Acknowledgements	1
Foreword	3
1. Plans, Plans	7
2. Who Turned on Our Heart?	9
3. Are You Treading Water?	15
4. Can't Keep Up?	19
5. The Long Midnight	21
6. Who in The World are You?	25
7. Never Lose Sight	29
8. For the Love of Mom	33
9. Bad COVID Hair Day	39
10. Closing a Chapter	43
11. "I Wonder What She Really Thinks"	47
12. The Final Music of George Floyd	51
13. The Wonder of Today and The Wonderboy	55
14. On the Other Side of the Knife	59

15.	Take the Plunge!	65
16.	Sow, Tend, Reap	69
17.	Running with Purpose	73
18.	Go Ahead and Flush!	77
19.	The Power of Giving Thanks	81
20.	Commitment During Calamity	87
21.	The New Look in Healthcare	91
22.	It's Heating Up Around Here	95
23.	How Can You Be Mad at This Face?	99
24.	Lamenting the Holidays	103
25.	Tired of Being Afraid?	107
26.	One Last Look at 2020	111
27.	On Turning 15	115
28.	When the Streets are Empty	119
29.	It's a Real Shame	123
30.	Time, Love, and Tenderness	127
31.	Thank You Saint Valentinus for the Love	131
32.	Riding the Wave	135
References		139
Additional Resources		143

For my husband, Thomas,
the writer who has inspired me to write

Acknowledgements

The stories from the global COVID-19 pandemic are never about just one person. Through the long midnight of the pandemic, each story is part of a larger shared journey. I have been privileged to be part of a special community which now includes you as you read.

I want to thank the many people who have contributed to helping me tell some of my own story as a health worker, mother, daughter, wife, and friend. Many of my Facebook friends have encouraged me regularly as I have posted blogs with my reflections and experiences during the pandemic. Thank you.

A special shout-out to my colleagues at St. Joseph's Hospital in Hamilton, ON, for being part of my story (and many of them as regular readers of my weekly blogs). Together, we have walked and served together during arguably the most challenging period of our careers. My friend and mentor Dr. Susan Ellis as Chief of Obstetrics/Gynecology at St. Joseph's has encouraged all of us health workers to provide the best and safest care we can during the pandemic.

My writing friends Patricia Paddey, Karen Stiller, Ruth Ann Bos, Denise Lodde Roberts and editor Krysia P. Lear have provided guidance and editing skills which have been greatly appreciated.

Global medical colleagues like Drs. Eve Nakabembe, Justus Barageine, Florence Mirembe and Pius Okong have always inspired me with their determination to provide life-saving maternal health care despite minimal support and significant risk to their own personal risk.

My thanks to the team from Friesen Publishing, including Brianne and the design team.

Most valued are my family members who have played such a large role in my story, especially my children, Liz, Jon and Hannah, and my parents, Gerald and Marg Chamberlain. Even when these loved ones experienced a potential COVID-19 exposure because of my work at the hospital, they cheered me on. I will always be grateful.

And finally, I am most thankful to my husband, Thomas Froese. His support, counsel, and encouragement have been a rock for me in this long midnight season, as well as over the 20 years of our marriage.

Dr. Jean Chamberlain-Froese

Foreword

I've long admired the work and witness of Dr. Jean Chamberlain-Froese, founder of Save the Mothers, the organization whose mission is to equip professionals in developing countries to improve the health of mothers and babies. To me, her work seemed like a model of a Christian life in service – to love God by saving the lives of mothers and their babies in Majority World countries.

With this book Dr. Jean does another kind of healing work. That is the healing that comes from sharing our true stories. Writer Anne Lamott says that "our stories are medicine." By telling the truth about our lives – the sometimes messy, wonderful, painful, joyful truth – we help to heal each other.

Our stories connect what other things can divide. Stories, honestly and well-told, build bridges, so we can understand and befriend each other and point each other to our loving God. Plus, I'm nosey, so it was fun to read a little bit about the daily life of a doctor living through COVID-19.

What you're holding in your hands is a glimpse of how Jean – doctor, mother, daughter, and wife (also, owner of a naughty puppy) – experienced her daily, personal, and professional life during the pandemic. It is a spiritual diary of sorts; a chronicle of a time we all shared together, yet dramatically apart. These stories and reflections will do their good work of connecting you with Jean, and with each other.

When Jean writes about standing alone in a late night, socially distanced line-up for take-out coffee during her shift as an obstetrician/gynecologist, for example, you catch a glimpse of a life and work that might be different from your own, but you will also recognize the feeling behind the story.

Simply put, the pandemic was a very weird time.

Jean helpfully wrote her way through it, and was able to see God in it, because of her knowledge of scripture, her experience of living through other rough times in sometimes rough places, and her long devotion to Jesus.

The life work of Jean Chamberlain-Froese is to be a healer. That's how God has used her and uses her still. This book is another expression of it that readers will welcome.

Karen Stiller is author of *The Minister's Wife* and a senior editor of *Faith Today* magazine.

March 18, 2020

1. Plans, Plans

It's March 18, 2020. There's not a person reading this post today whose plans haven't been drastically altered in the past five days by COVID-19. The announcements of upcoming concerts and meetings, reminders of appointments, and schedules of school activities all seem incredibly irrelevant and attached to a world far away. Most events are cancelled.

Hearing my kids worry about not graduating from elementary school, losing their summer break, and if the world will ever be as they knew it—it's emotionally exhausting. I've given up on my Freedom 55 birthday party, scheduled to happen in just over a week. Kelly Williams Scott, my childhood friend, and I will have to simply FaceTime to celebrate together. We have to keep our distance!

In a world where my plans have long been scheduled into my Outlook calendar, this new world seems destabilizing. But then I was reminded of the great scheduler—the One who made the Big Dipper star pattern that I was gazing at the other evening. His words of calm and encouragement bring hope when the news tells us the increasing count for COVID-19. "For I know the plans I have for you," declares the Lord. "Plans to prosper you and not to harm you, plans to give you hope and a future" (Jeremiah 29:11, NIV).[1] Of course, I prefer that those plans are without discomfort or suffering. But we are warned that we will have challenges and pain in this life: knowing the One who has overcome all of these, gives each us the strength and hope to know that the purpose of our lives, is greater than any schedule, event or job. It gives me the stability to walk one step at a time today, and not feel drowned by threats of a tsunami in the future.

Dear Friends: My hope and prayer are that you will be secure within the arms of Christ and the bigger purpose and plan that He has for you. In the meantime, keep washing your hands and watching out for the vulnerable in your community.

Dr. Jean

Adobe Images

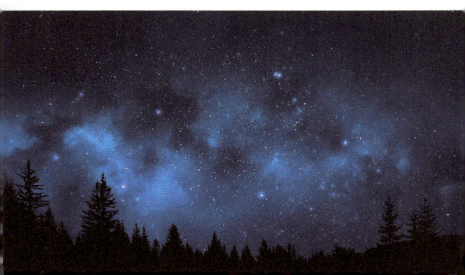

March 22, 2020

2. Who Turned on Our Heart?

Here's a question: Who turned on your heart this morning? Not who or what motivated you or even attracted you, but literally, how did your heart start beating? Of course, it was beating all night. We never give it a second thought. Now I know some bright health worker will point out that some patients have an implanted defibrillator that restarts their heart when it stops, but those individuals are the exception. For most of us, our heart beats all night and is still pumping in the morning.

In this time of uncertainty and change, I hope that when you wake up tomorrow morning, you take a brief moment to thank God for a beating heart—that He has kept that electrical pump going all night. These days, our hearts all feel strained, especially those of our elderly friends and family, who are being separated from loved ones for their own safety.

Dr. Jean Chamberlain-Froese

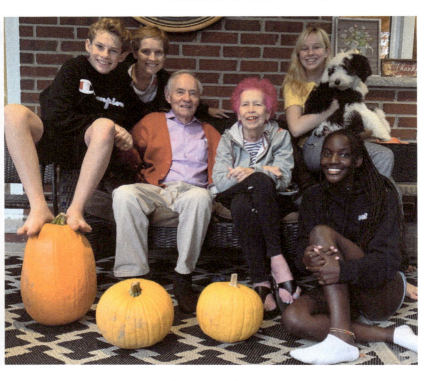

My parents (centre), Gerald and Margaret Chamberlain, surrounded by our children Jon, Hannah, and Liz (far right) —the separation from grandparents seemed endless during the pandemic restrictions. This photo was taken later in the pandemic when small outside gatherings were permitted.

I was saddened to learn yesterday that my parents can't leave their seniors' residence here in Dundas due to the fear of COVID-19 outbreaks in the region. I've never lived so close to my parents, yet I can't even visit them or take them to my home. It brought tears to my eyes.

Our Long Midnight

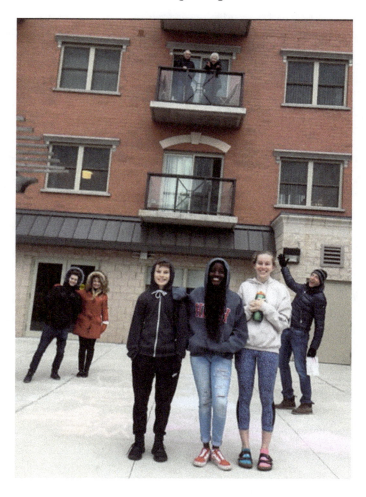

Balcony visits only with Dad and Mom Chamberlain (on balcony) with family members (left to right); nephew Matt and my sister Cathy Eeuwes; our children Jon, Hannah, Liz with my husband, Thomas Froese.

My dear friends Sam and Gloria Williams had to have a window visit with their great granddaughter. It all seems so unnatural. Yet in the instability and uncertainty, many of us are seeing the care and generosity of others and we're stopping to see and appreciate the small things of life, like simply giving someone a hug!

I remember working for a short time in a rural and somewhat unstable area of Democratic Republic of Congo in East Africa. I was 32-weeks pregnant and working with Drs. Philip and Nancy Wood. Each night, Philip listened to the shortwave radio to hear where the rebels were stationed. It was a tense time for us. But I couldn't help but think of the pregnant Congolese women who were there—they lived permanently in that instability.

When I arrived later in Canada to deliver my baby, I had a new sense of thankfulness for the personal safety we have here in North America. I understood more deeply how insecurity so significantly affects young moms and their babies. I'm certain many of my Syrian refugee mothers could tell me stories like those of the Congolese women of not being able to get to a hospital in time to receive care for themselves or their babies.

In this time of instability, we all are experiencing the loss of personal freedoms and choices, and some are losing loved ones or their health. As we walk through this time, we will be become different people on the other side.

One movie that I've seen explores how we can be changed people is the Jesus Film[a] —it's available in hundreds of languages. It's worth watching and will give you

---

a   The film "Jesus," https://www.jesusfilm.org/watch/jesus

an insightful look at the life and challenging moments in the life of Jesus.

Dear Friends: My prayer is that as you wake up in the morning, that you remember the One who has kept your heart beating all night. Give a word of thanks and spend some of your newfound quiet moments exploring His purpose for your life. Safety and peace to each of you.

Dr. Jean

April 5, 2020

3. Are You Treading Water?

Are you treading water? Probably not, as all public pools are closed and few of us have an indoor, private pool. I always hated treading water when I was a kid. My dear mom, Marg Chamberlain, made sure that each of us could swim and tread water. Yes, we completed the classic life-saving Red Cross lessons, and, worst of all, we suffered through them in a freezing cold Ontario lake at Camp Mini-Yo-We near Huntsville in Muskoka, north of Toronto.

Treading water was one of those burdensome skills that have to be mastered as a part of swimming lessons. The motion of your arms and legs underwater keeps your lower body from sinking to the bottom of the lake. The worst part about treading water was that despite all the effort it took to do it properly, you went nowhere. After 10 minutes and a lot of energy, especially in cold lake, you started and stopped in the same spot!

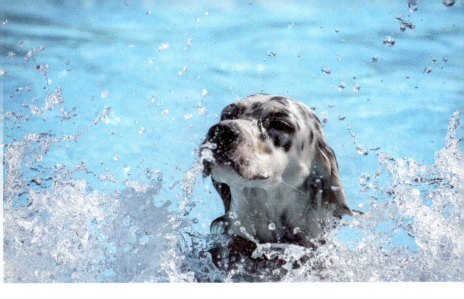

Adobe Images

But the goal of treading water was not to go places, it was to keep your head above the water, to stay alive—especially in situations such as being dumped out of a boat or finding yourself too far from shore and unable to swim. You would call on your skill to tread water until someone rescued you or you could swim further. The goal of treading water was life, not progress.

So, I come back to my original question: How many of us feel like we are treading water, just keeping our heads above the level of the water right now? The key is that you are treading. You are "walking in the water" with all of your strength and keeping your head afloat.

I recently spoke with several East African friends who live very close to survival level, with no bank account or other savings to count on. Before COVID-19, many already lived day to day. If they don't make money today, they don't eat tomorrow. That's how close it is for them all

Our Long Midnight

the time. The reality of COVID-19 has only brought the water level higher. They can almost taste the water now.

But I've also learned some lessons from my East African friends about living today where I am, and not in the future (including tomorrow). Those lessons are well described by Sarah Young[2], a writer whose personal suffering has brought her closer to God in uncertain times. In one of her posts, she writes, 1) "Do not linger in the future, because anxieties sprout up ..."; 2) "Remember the promise of God's continual presence ... This mental discipline does not come easily."

Many of us heard Queen Elizabeth II speak to her nation and the world today about COVID (I hope I look that good at 93 years of age!). She reflected on the practical discipline of fighting this disease; there is also a discipline in maintaining our own mental and spiritual health. Sarah's reflections two guiding principles for maintaining our mental and spiritual health. These disciplines will help us to effectively tread water during these challenging times. We may not feel like we are making progress, but we are! In addition to staying alive (with our head above water), we are gaining strength and stamina that we would never have acquired during our "normal" days and experience.

And as Jesus, the One whose suffering we remember at the end of this Holy Week, said himself, "Do not worry about tomorrow. For tomorrow will worry about its own things. Sufficient for the day is its own trouble" (Matthew

6:34). If you want to learn more, take some time to see the acclaimed film *Risen*.[b]

Treading water. Not lingering in the future. Remembering God's presence. Learning new things. These are the disciplines for each of us: whether at home or returning to the hospital / essential service tomorrow.

Dear Friends: My prayer for you is that as we long for Easter Sunday, this week, Holy Week, be a time that is full of meaning and courage, even in the midst of the rising waters. Easter Sunday is that day to celebrate that Jesus was able to rise up from His own death and suffering to give us hope in ours.

Dr. Jean

---

b The film "Risen" available at https://www.youtube.com/watch?v=tgM1WGFTtjE

April 13, 2020

4. Can't Keep Up?

What are the Froese Five kids doing with their Freedom 55 Mother on Easter Weekend? My 16-year-old, Liz, is a committed runner and wants to get some exercise with her aging mom (and I'm all for it, just probably not running as far as she is hoping). My Ugandan daughter, Hannah, and son Jon are recruited to join the training. Close to our home is a lovely park with a cemetery at the far end. During the COVID-19 crisis with its multiple restrictions to public places, the park is seeing more daily visitors than usual. We all easily keep our six feet distance from others. But strangely, after circling the park numerous times, the cemetery seems like an attractive place to continue our several kilometres run.

By now, I'm not as energetic (and please know that we had to run up a flight of stairs to reach the cemetery). I remind myself that I can no longer keep up with my athletic kids. I somehow stumble into the graveyard, slowing my pace as my teammates race ahead. As I watch my three teens run on the designated roads through this nearly two-century-old cemetery, I can't help but see a little piece of Easter in this quiet place. Death has been overtaken by life in the six strong legs of my children as they pass the tombstones. And that new life embraces the world.

I'm reminded that even though this is a place of death for many, God can bring new and unexpected life and joy to this place. I can see the joy in my children's faces.

And by the way, Thom has already purchased our couple's plot at the lower end of this cemetery. I have my place secured. The reality, though, is that I won't really be in that grave anyway. My spirit will be with the One who was resurrected on this Easter morning. And that is the hope of anyone who embraces the power of the Easter story.

Dear Friends: My prayer is that it will change your lives, also.

Dr. Jean

April 20, 2020

5. The Long Midnight

As an obstetrician, I find myself often working at midnight. I guess it comes with the job. I don't know a lot of healthcare workers who love the night shift. It always seems kind of sombre and maybe it's unnatural to be up at that hour, sometimes making important decisions that can save (or lose) a life. Of course, the babies see it differently and come whenever they decide. I've always appreciated a comment from a colleague of mine: "No matter how tired you are (in the middle of the night), just remember, the morning is coming and there will be someone there to relieve you!" That reminder does bring some hope when your third cup of coffee just isn't doing it for you.

By the way, our Tim Horton's in the hospital closes at 11:30 p.m. so there's always a big rush to get our final coffee of the night. Interestingly, during COVID-19, I have never seen the lines so sparse. It's all because of the "no visitor" hospital policy. I have to say, it does cut back on Timmy's lines—and of course, we are all standing two metres apart in our hospital greens!

In my effort to keep myself at least a little healthier these days, I've been exercising and listening to music. One song that has struck me is the "Midnight" by Rita Springer. I love the picture that it paints: God does not wait until the sunrise to help us. He bursts through at midnight.

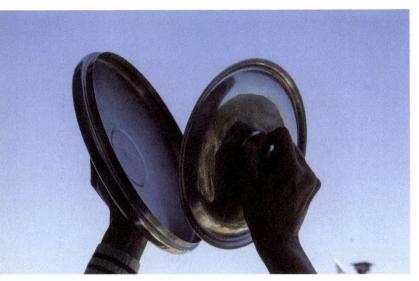

Hospital neighbours clanged pot lids at 7:30 p.m. to thank frontline workers.
Adobe Images

For many people right now, midnight feels very long. It seems like an eternity before the sunrise—before there is help coming. I spoke with a colleague from Uganda today, and her stories of the situation mothers and their newborns are heartbreaking. (And as a frontline health worker, thank all of you who continue to support our efforts here).

After speaking with my Ugandan colleague, I couldn't help but think that in this midnight time God is calling out to us as our father. It may seem like a paradox, but it is as if He is trying to get our attention when there's so much less distraction and activity swirling around us.

Midnights can happen at any stage in our lives. In the early days of late 2009 after Hannah, joined our family from her orphanage in, She would burst into tears when Dorothy, our Ugandan nanny, left for the day. Dorothy reminded her of the caregivers at the orphanage. Hannah would cry out "Mama" and reach for Dorothy. Of course, I was holding back tears behind her—I was her mommy, but she didn't yet believe that in her little four-year-old heart. I could hardly blame her.

Recently, for my Freedom 55 birthday, Hannah wrote the most beautiful card describing how our relationship has grown to be so meaningful to her—that she is so glad that I am her mother. I couldn't hold back the tears, again!

It reminded me that people sometimes want to stay where it is comfortable, with what they know. But if they'll let go, a new life, which is greater than they could ever imagine, is just ahead.

I see God's heart breaking as He longs to hold us as our father and wipe our tears as a mother. I hope that during any long midnight, we will be willing to hear His true message—not the meaningless and inaccurate ideas about Him that sometimes come from nonreligious and religious individuals. Rather, the one that comes through the message and life of Christ.

Dear Friends: This week, I pray that even if you do not see any light in your midnight, you will take a moment to listen to this song and be reminded of the one who is with you at this difficult time. "Midnight"[3] by Rita Springer—her song to our Father, who has "perfect timing."

Dr. Jean

April 26, 2020

6. Who in The World are You?

You can't live in a household of teenagers without being reminded of the many years that we all spend trying to figure out who we are. What's the image we are trying to portray? Who are the friends we want to hang around with and the standard old question, "What do you want to be when you grow up?"

There's a lot of musing in our family about "six-pack abs" — Liz has a training program if you are at all interested. We can chuckle a bit at that, but regardless of our stage of life, people can still be seen to be pushing for centre stage. They're just a little less obvious than a teenager standing in front of the mirror admiring their physique or muscles.

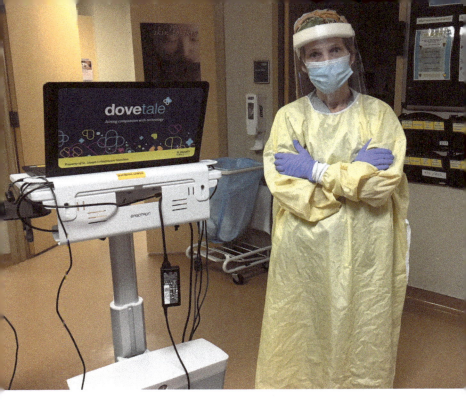

Dr. Jean Chamberlain-Froese is ready for action in her personal protection equipment (PPE).

I had a bit of a centre stage experience this past week when we put together a video about delivering a baby during COVID-19. I certainly didn't have to worry about my make-up or hair. I was all decked out in a mask and O.R. hat—it's really difficult to see my mascara. We joked about it being "Jollywood" (meaning it was filmed at St. Joe's, Hamilton). The video was intended to help people understand a little bit more about the fears and concerns of pregnant women at this time.[c]

---

c https://www.youtube.com/watch?v=cduSDQdLTQM&t=4s

Even after a long day of caring for moms and trying to make a difference, I am reminded that even in the middle of this global catastrophe, I can relax in who I really am. I can rest in the fact that I am the child of One who loves me regardless of my imperfections or anything good that I may be able to do.

Those of you who know me, know I love music: both listening and playing. Even when Liz was a little girl, I had her learning to play the piano. The other two kids followed suit. Music brings a lot of joy and a reminder of what is so central in our lives. Chris Tomlin sings about being loved by God, "a good, good Father."[4] Hearing that brings a smile to my face as I drive home from the hospital. I am loved by my Father. That's who I am. That's who you are.

And our Father wants us to love others as Christ loved us. That doesn't mean living with a happy, plastic face, but rather caring deeply for people in both their strengths and weaknesses. It means being honestly happy when others succeed even if it might leave me behind. It, also means loving them in their vulnerabilities. I was thinking about friends who work at places like the Salvation Army or Teen Challenge—helping people who are caught in addiction. These organizations and their staff do not just give these vulnerable people something to eat but also give them the tough love they need to fight against the habits that are harming them.

Jesus loved the people he rubbed shoulders with. He didn't let his friend Peter just forget about denying him three times. Rather, He gave Peter the three chances to reaffirm his love for Jesus.

Understanding who we really are —once we have received that gift of adoption into God's family—gives us not only incredible peace but also a sense of who we are regardless of the circumstances. It gives us the power to really love others into being the people that God wants them to be.

Dear Friends: May the truth of who you are, and how much you are loved by God through the incredible gift of Jesus Christ, bring you hope and peace this week in whatever you will face.

Dr. Jean

May 3, 2020

7. Never Lose Sight

I get a lot of inspiration from marathon runners, but I will never be one. That was determined early in my athletic career. I was more likely to get the "inspirational" award than the "most valuable player." The closest thing I got to running a marathon was a short 10-kilometre route with a young colleague, Dr. Laura Hopkins.

Dr. Hopkins is now a talented gynecological oncologist in Saskatoon. In the mid-nineties, she and I would regularly run in Dundas, Ontario, where she lived. I was living in downtown Hamilton. One big empty field we ran by is now the site of the seniors' residence where my parents live. I would return from my run with Laura, huffing and puffing. I always looked forward to the end of the 10 kilometres: the sense of accomplishment, and the chat and rest and relaxation to follow.

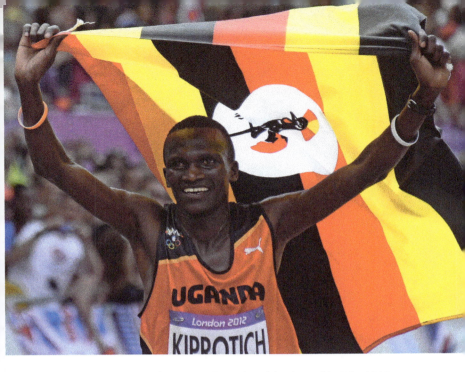

Ugandan marathoner Stephen Kiprotich wins gold at the 2012 London Olympics.
AFP, New Vision Uganda

My small efforts were only a small shadow of those of real marathoners. I'm amazed at the courage and persistence of individuals like Stephen Kiprotich, who achieved one of Uganda's greatest national moments. Stephen Kiprotich is now a household name in Uganda. He won the 2012 Olympic marathon in London. This Olympic gold medalist, the youngest of seven children, never finished high school and came from a poor rural area of Eastern Uganda. Stephen had learned how to see the end of the marathon. The end of the 42.19 kilometres. When he first started the race, he was surrounded by hundreds of others, and with each pace, his body would remind him of the pain of the journey as his tired feet hit the asphalt over and over. With each of the 55,374 steps that he took, he always centred on the fact that there was an end. He wasn't running to only arbitrarily stop in downtown London. Having a destination gave him hope so he could keep going and finish the race at the front of the line.

My children had the privilege of meeting him when he came to visit their international school in Uganda.

By the way, I witnessed some real live hope this week at my Hamilton hospital. I had the privilege of helping to deliver a patient of mine who had suffered six consecutive miscarriages with no living children. She was well into her child-bearing years, but this past week, she delivered her first living baby—a beautiful boy. I don't think there was a dry eye in the birthing room. She had run a marathon and never lost sight of the end.

Our lives are a lot like a marathon. Right now, our feet are feeling every pushback from the hard pavement. The pain of the "right now" can obscure the finish line. Despite the incredible discomfort and our bodies crying out to stop, we can never lose sight of the finish line.

But, unlike a physical marathon, the hope of getting to the end of the marathon of life does not depend on our abilities, planning, or stamina. It's centred on who we are and the one who is running with us. In "No Longer Slaves," which he recorded at Harding Prison, Nashville, Zach Williams sings "I'm no longer a slave to fear." And affirms that he is a "child of God."[d] I hope you take a moment to listen.

Prior to COVID-19, it was easy to dismiss that song's relevance. But within a short time, it seems that many of us are living in a prison of fear, a lonely place that makes us feel without purpose or meaningful end.

How do we reach that meaningful finish line? I gained that hope I realized that I needed someone to run with, someone who had run the race before me and successfully finished his own marathon: Jesus Christ. The irony is that He knew that His would end in severe suffering and loneliness. His victory, the prize He obtained, allowed us to receive the adoption papers of being called the children of God. Christ's life, His death and resurrection, bought each of us those eternal papers and forever changed who we are.

It means that at the end of each of our own marathons, we will enjoy an incredible celebration that lasts forever with Christ, the ultimate marathoner. I hope you will invite Him to run with you today. Your journey will never be the same. Mine hasn't.

Dear Friends: As your toes get crushed by stones on the road this week, when your ankle turns and sweat is pouring down your face, remember to never lose sight of the finish line and the One who runs beside you.

Dr. Jean

---

d   "No Longer Slaves" (2018) by Zach Williams: https://www.youtube.com/watch?v=bDnA_coA168

May 10, 2020

8. For the Love of Mom

Usually on Mother's Day weekend—when there is no global pandemic—I'm busy with the Save the Mothers' walk, which helps raise support for vulnerable mothers in East Africa. This year on the eve and early morning of Mother's Day, I had the privilege of delivering three new moms and was one of the first to wish them a Happy Mother's Day.

But my thoughts as I reflect on this Mother's Day are not on these new moms or even those who are bereaved. I am thinking about a senior mom, who has spent a lifetime raising children and is now cared for by those children. I'll call her Vera. She's over 90 and was admitted the other day to my hospital with a serious gynecological complication. When I met her on the ward, she was alone, confused, and fighting back tears.

Because of pandemic restrictions, her sons couldn't visit her. She had no phone and sat alone in the hospital bed, with a commode parked beside her. When I took over care, I used my mobile phone to call her son. I expected a man in his 50s. He was 71 and caring for a very ill wife. His elderly mother (now my patient) normally lived in the house beside him. I could hear the fear in his voice as we talked about whether his mother needed surgery or some other treatment.

He spoke to her in her own Eastern European language and would complete his paragraph saying, "I love you mom!" I don't know why he would always say it in English. He said it about four times, maybe for my benefit so that I would know that this dear woman was the mother of someone. That someone was a man of 71 years.

Later that day, the medical team was relieved to finally conclude that her situation was not so acute. She would not require surgery, an intervention that is pretty tough on anyone let alone a woman in her 90s. For many hours, Vera had been kept "NPO"— "nothing per os," aka nothing to eat, in anticipation of surgery. When she heard the good news, she wouldn't have surgery, her attention immediately went to her forfeited morning coffee.

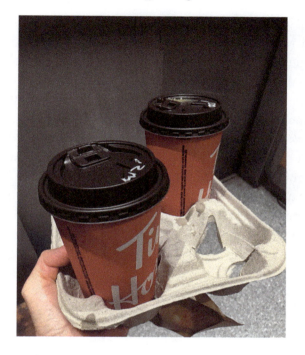

Dr. Jean taking coffee to the floor for the 90 year old patient.

Unfortunately, she had missed the hospital order for lunch. Quite happy to have a quick coffee break myself, I ran down to our faithful Timmy's and grabbed coffee for the two of us. Her eyes widened when I walked in the room with her coffee in hand. Her morning would be okay.

This brief interaction reminded me that no matter how old we are, we love our moms as well as the "mothers" in our lives. My heart goes out to the many people who couldn't see their moms this Mother's Day or whose moms were alone for medical or quarantine reasons. I pray that somehow, through a coffee or the face of a friendly health worker, they will know how much they are loved.

I do have some happy news that Vera should soon be out of the hospital. She has a bit of a rough road ahead but has two wonderful sons who will continue to care for her to the best of their ability regardless of how little or much time she has ahead on this planet.

We all thank God for the mothers and mother figures in our lives and send out a big shout-out to them for a lifetime of service and care. On Sunday we had an outdoor visit with my mom. We stood on the sidewalk, peering up at her, where she stood beside my dad on their third-floor balcony.

As we try to care for mothers in these challenging days, let us also remember the other vulnerable mothers who, during this global economic collapse, not only face the dangers of delivering in places with few resources but may not even be able to reach a healthcare facility. All public transport in Uganda has been closed for weeks. It was the only means for many mothers to reach hospitals. You can't walk 10 kilometres to the nearest health facility while in labour. Already, these women's chances of dying from pregnancy complications were at least 50 times higher than for women in Canada. Now their lifeline to health care facilities is gone.

Do take a minute to remember and pray for these women. And as you feel led, please support organizations like Save the Mothers who are coming up with creative ways to help needy women and their babies.

Dear Friends: Remember the mother(s) in your lives, and for those of you who are mothers and mother figures to others, we thank you for your love, patience, and smile!

Dr. Jean

May 17, 2020

9. Bad COVID Hair Day

I saw our Canadian prime minister tonight on the television news, his hair blown about by the wind, and for the first time, I can honestly say that I felt sorry for him. I pitied that he didn't have two teenage daughters to help him with his rather unruly hair. I've been fighting the same battle myself recently as I'm sure many of you have. I finally got desperate and picked up some hair dye from a pharmacy and then sharpened my best pair of scissors. I encouraged my daughters to go online and augment their hairdressing skills. After all, they are doing lots of online learning these days. Why not work on their mother's mop?

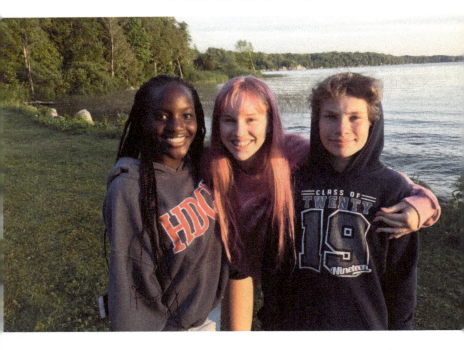

Each of my kids (Hannah, Liz, Jon) did something different with their hair during the COVID-19 pandemic.

The process was all rather fun and, quite frankly, an opportunity to see the strengths of both girls. Hannah definitely had the edge with the hair colouring. I've been highlighting my hair for several years, but yesterday was my first attempt at it without professional help. Liz shone in sculpting my hair. Thomas, my husband, was so impressed that he was begging the girls for a clip at the end of the day.

I have to admit that having unruly hair makes me feel a bit unsettled. I guess we all have our own gauge for assessing our comfort with our appearance and clothing. One of my Ugandan friends told me that she would much rather go to bed hungry and know that she had something nice to wear in the morning than to eat and have nothing attractive to wear the next day. I think I can understand where she's coming from.

Even in the best of times, we are pulled and pushed in life in so many ways. But this global pandemic has sharpened our sensitivity to the strength of these forces. Many in our generation have never experienced such powerful upheavals in their everyday life. Those who have lived through world wars or civil wars have a tasted this. It has thrown off our stability: our balance. We struggle to regain our equilibrium to maintain hope for the future despite the disappointments of daily life.

Death can be a tremendous push in our lives. I reflect on two funerals this week that I was connected to. One was for a young man who left his wife and two little children, having died suddenly, with so many questions yet to be answered. The other being that of the mother of a friend, a person who has touched countless individuals. Few could attend her service in person, yet her well-lived life was celebrated in a beautiful way

Life also has its pulls and pushes. Ask any young mother in my waiting room: she has never slept so little, never worked so hard, and never felt her emotions so out of whack. I've seen it all in my practice and felt that way as a young mom myself.

Equilibrium. It's the steadiness of keeping both sides balanced: the pulls and pushes of life. Even the once simple tasks, like of keeping one's hair well groomed, can seem beyond reach. I find myself unable to maintain life's balance when my strength is exhausted and my usual go-tos are gone. It's then that I'm reminded of Jesus' wonderful invitation to "Come to me all who are weary and heavy laden and I will give you rest" (Matthew 11:28, NIV). Jesus gives us rest, not just in the times of peace but when the pulls and the pushes in life are overwhelming, when the centre of our hearts and souls are strained with pain. As I drive to the hospital each day and ponder the uncertain times and days ahead, I have found no other effective lasting source of peace.

Dear Friends: As we face the happenings of this next week, whether they're an opening or closing, joy or disappointment, new life, or loss of life, let us remember that timeless invitation from Jesus Christ. He experienced incredible pain and suffering, rejection, and humiliation knowing that through his life and death, he could offer us rest. Rest for now and rest for eternity.

Dr. Jean

May 23, 2020

10. Closing a Chapter

I'll be first to admit it. I'm a terrible sentimentalist who sobs at the sappiest of movies and should be the least likely to be chosen to speak at a funeral. So, I wondered what I was going to do yesterday while helping to clean out my parents' former home in Toronto. The sale of my parents' condo townhouse closes this weekend. It represented the final page in a chapter. They have already moved to a seniors' residence in Dundas just minutes from my front door. I had volunteered to help with final cleaning.

It's a closing chapter in my parents' and our family's lives: their 10 years in a great place served my folks very well in their senior years. We, the Froese Family Five, would stay there for weeks at a time in our annual transitions from Uganda to Canada. The halls are filled with memories.

A lot of chapters have closed for many people in the last few months. For some, the closings were happy, but for the majority, the chapters brought more tears than smiles.

Our newspapers are full of these kinds of stories. Thom recently wrote about the desperate situation in Uganda.[e]

For our Muslim friends, today, May 24, represents the end of Ramadan and the start of Eid al-Fitr, so Happy Eid to all our friends who are celebrating. I remember living in Yemen and feeling the palpable relief experienced by my Yemeni neighbours at the end of Ramadan, the month of fasting. It can be a long chapter, fasting, especially during hot seasons when the days are long.

Meanwhile, children in Ontario were excited and saddened to learn that their school year is closed for in-person learning for the remainder of the school year. No doubt, some parents wept! Many camps like Ontario Pioneer and Mini-Yo-We were forced to cancel their plans for overnight camps this summer, closing a chapter of providing over 70 years of non-stop annual camping for children.

What do we do with these closed chapters? You can no doubt name another ten. For me, my hope comes from resting in the One who is writing your and my chapters, knowing that He is the great author of our lives. I get a lot of comfort from the verse in Psalms, which reads: *"Your eyes saw my unformed body. All the days ordained for me were written in your book before one of them came to be"* (Psalm 139:16)

---

[e] "Pandemic wolf stalks developing world" by Thomas Froese. The Hamilton Spectator: Saturday, May 23, 2020: https://www.thomasfroese.com/tag/pandemic-in-developing-world/

In a great mystery that is beyond my finite understanding of this planet, there is One who knows each of our days. He knows all the chapters. He knew which door would close behind us or our families and He knew which ones would open. They may be even quiet chapters of rest or perceived inactivity, chapters of frustration and palpable grief, but He knows. Even our last chapter here on Earth is only the introduction to an eternal chapter of enjoying His presence.

I've had the privilege of writing two books about global maternal health, *Where Have all the Mothers Gone?* and the second, co-authored with my talented friend Patricia Paddey, *Game Changers*. Thom and I found a copy of both books yesterday as we cleaned out mom and dad's place. Those books both had beginnings and endings. The author of our lives has promised no end to our final chapter.

This reminds me of a song that I have loved since my childhood. It's a ballad or hymn by the Chicago-based lawyer Horatio Goertner Spafford, "It Is Well with My Soul." Spafford composed it as he sailed over the place in the Atlantic Ocean where his four daughters had drowned in a shipping accident in 1873. He had lost much of his livelihood in the great Chicago fire in 1871, and now all his remaining beloved children had perished in the ocean. He didn't understand why it was happening, and he would have no idea that his simple heart song would impact so many lives over many decades. With tears in his eyes as he passed the accident's tragic location, he could whisper, "It is well with my soul."[5] Here is the first verse of that song (in modern English):

> When peace, like a river, attends my way,
> When sorrows like sea billows roll;
> Whatever my lot, you have taught me to say,
> It is well, it is well with my soul.

Dear Friends: I pray that you will also know that the chapters of your life are not random and without hope. It's true that, on this big globe your chapters may be rainy at times, peaceful at others, and tragic at the worst of times. But there is One who sees each chapter and waits intently for that final one that leads us into our eternity with Him if we have chosen to embrace Him.

Dr. Jean

May 31, 2020

11. "I Wonder What She Really Thinks"

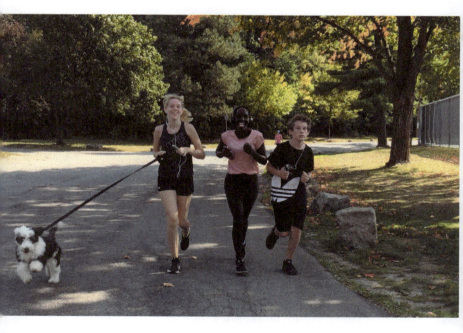

Liz, Hannah and Jon running in a local park with Gracie trying to keep up.

Most mornings I forget that my younger daughter Hannah is African, that she came from the other side of the world, and that naturally she has beautiful ebony skin that shines on her muscular arms. I simply forget. But she doesn't because her greater world doesn't let her.

While she was walking with her fair-skinned siblings in the neighbourhood recently during the COVID-19 pandemic, Hannah, an inquiring policewoman asked, "Are you all from one family?" I don't think the police officer was being racist; she was just doing her job, but for Hannah, it was a reminder of an assumed difference.

I delivered six beautiful babies last night. They came from various racial backgrounds and circumstances. Some were born to teens and others to older women with more life experience and financial resources. With each of those babies, we waited for them to let out that first big cry: to let the world know that they've arrived. Each one was celebrated and treated with tremendous and equal worth.

How does that status change over time?

As we fight to stamp out racism around the globe and around the corner, we need to work from common ground: the equal value of each human being. We need a foundation for our uniqueness and value that comes from somewhere that doesn't shift with changing governments and philosophies.

There are many theories and ideas, but for me, the most logical one comes from the life and words of Jesus Christ. He reminded each of us of our worth as creations of God. We weren't random happenings. He reached out to the victims of prejudice in his lifetime, specifically, a marginalized racial group called the "Samaritans," people who experienced palpable racism and discrimination. Jesus was also counter cultural, speaking respectfully with women, who in his generation, were not even considered reliable in a court of law.

My husband, Thom, showed the family a video by Tyler Merritt, "Before You Call the Cops," In this monologue, this "proud Black" actor, confident of who he is, settled in his knowledge of being a creation of God, compellingly introduces himself and his family. In it, he expresses the daily hurt he experiences as a result of racism. Take a moment to look here.[f]

I wondered about Hannah's reflection to Tyler's soliloquy. As usual, she didn't say a lot, but expressed herself non-verbally in agreement with his concerns about the racism he experiences. My hope is that she will always know she is: A loved child appreciated for who she is as an individual. That she receives her value not only from us, but also from her Creator and the One who longs to be all that she needs, even in moments of difficulty and prejudice.

As a white Canadian woman, I have rarely experienced significant prejudice and racism. The worst I can recall is being turned away at a Yemeni airport because I was a woman. My husband was allowed to enter it and greet the international visiting professor, whom I had invited, while I was forced to wait elsewhere because of my gender.

---

f   "Before You Call the Cops" (2018). Tyler Merritt Project: https://www.youtube.com/watch?v=wKeITMzMn7w

It boiled my blood for a minute, but I've never had my blood shed as a victim of racism.

So, I'll let Hannah have the final word here. Borrowing from some popular songs, in a recent English school assignment she strung together about her views of racism: "If you can't see my colour, you can't see me. We're more beautiful when we come together. Let's all fight for each other instead of against each other. Let's stand in unity."

Dear Friends: I pray that you will know Christ's peace and plan for your life: to recognize His love for you and each person that walks this planet regardless of the shoes they wear.

Dr. Jean

June 14, 2020

12. The Final Music of George Floyd

I taught piano as a teen myself and later became entangled in helping my three children to acquire some musical abilities. Hats off to my three kids' piano teachers. I reap the benefits some evenings, listening to them sing and play with the honest inspiration and passion of teens.

It makes me think about music and the power of it. I wrote a surprise song for Thom when we got married, 19 years ago now. The song was called 'Surprised by Joy' and I played it for Thom for the first time at our wedding reception. I was still wearing my wedding gown. He tells me he had a tear in his eye. The power of music.

I often wonder how certain tones and words when strung together can create such a powerful impression. The combined impact is greater than the sum of the individual words or tones standing alone. The phenomenon has been the study of music sociologists for many years. The power of a song has moved many of us to tears at some time in our lives.

Speaking of music, probably like you, I've been learning about the life of George Floyd and reflecting on his recent funeral, which was filled with powerful music. George Floyd had a rough start in life, had bumps along the road, including some run-ins with the law. But he made conscious choices to embrace Christ and the path that Christ would want him to follow. That choice would lead him to new beginnings, even if in another state in America. Music was an important part of his life, and one medium through which he expressed his hope and faith.

It is only fitting that music was a central part of the memorial for his life. The four-hour service started off with the song gospel singer Andraé Crouch: "The Blood Will Never Lose Its Power." I remember hearing Andraé sing this gripping song when I was a child at my family's church, The Peoples Church, in Toronto. What a great name for a church: a reminder that it is a place for all peoples. Andraé wrote that song when he himself was only 15 years of age. Even in his early teens, Andraé understood the message and life of Jesus. Jesus' message has been a difficult one to embrace at various times in history, both for people in Jesus' own generation as well in ours. Jesus emphasized the need for each of us having a new beginning as human beings and the core need for forgiveness for ourselves and others. Jesus' power and impact came through Jesus himself—His death and resurrection—and not simply through his words or kind acts of healing.

We don't necessarily like to talk about blood these days. It's not really a coffee table conversation. But there's no life without the loss of blood. I've never attended a newborn delivery without the mother losing some blood.

Andraé's song describes the impact of Jesus' blood: "It soothes my doubts and calms my fears and it dries all my tears. The blood that gives me strength from day to day, it will never lose its power."[6]

Floyd had been leaning into the strength and power of Christ's love and forgiveness as he worked with youth in in Houston and later in security at the Salvation Army's Harbor Light Centre in Minneapolis. To understand Floyd's journey, we need to understand and acknowledge the new beginnings that he was experiencing because of his faith and assurance in Christ. Despite the many challenges He faced, He knew that He was loved, and it strengthened Him to love others, regardless of how they treated Him. As his friend Tiffany Cofield said, "I've come to believe that He was chosen. Only this could have happened to Him because of who He was and the amount of love that He had for people and that people had for Him."[7]

Dear Friends: My prayer is that we would know that song of Floyd's life, and that it will continue to be sung around the world for a very long time. They are powerful words with a tune that should never get out of our hearts and minds.

Dr. Jean

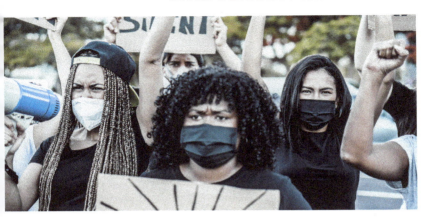

Women at a rally in memory of George Floyd, June 2020.
Adobe Images

July 14, 2020

13. The Wonder of Today and The Wonderboy

Tonight, as we sat around the dinner table playing one of my family's favourite games, "The UnGame," (a game of questions), I drew the card that asked: "What age group do you find most challenging to be around?" The kids were a bit surprised with my answer: Two-to-three-year-olds.

I love delivering babies and cooing over them with their young parents. But my strength probably isn't working full-time with two or three-year-old children in a daycare. Having said that, I am constantly amazed by the ability of young children to be fascinated by the little things around them. They insist on taking the time to admire the flowers, the colours, and even the bugs.

Young children love to stand in front of our home where a small creek passes through our property. With their parents waiting patiently at their sides, the little ones admire the running water. Like those children, as I am captivated by nature, and take time to gaze at the silhouette of the Niagara Escarpment near our home or to admire the turtles crossing the road near the wildlife sanctuary by our home. I am reminded of the beautiful gift of nature and life right in front of me each day.

Recently, I have been caring, directly or indirectly, for younger women with significant gynecological cancers. Among them are new moms. I see how they treasure each day and find joy in it. It reminds me to stop each day and see the beauty in my children, the daily care given by my husband, the earnestness of my parents, and the concern of my neighbours, as wonderful gifts.

Speaking of the wonder of the day, I had the privilege of delivering a beautiful little girl today. The mom needed some special attention for a safe delivery, and we performed a caesarean section. But it was a special delivery also as it corresponds to my husband Thom's 55th birthday.

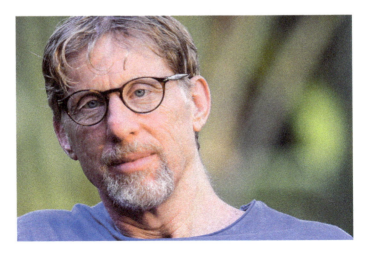

Thomas Froese celebrates 55 years of life.

Yes, the young Thomas Froese, who came to Canada as a child, is now 55. He finally caught up with his older wife. As it is, I see Thom as a bit of a Wonderboy with a story. He was a runaway, in a way, before he was born, having left Canada for Germany while still in his mother's womb. After birth he was later battled over in an international custody case, and cared for by extended family as a new immigrant to Canada. He learned a new language and way of life and eventually found his calling as a journalist, to be a voice to people of different backgrounds and beliefs for more than 30 years. His career has taken him to a variety of places on several continents, from locations like Yemen and Uganda, along with Canadian locales like Toronto, Hamilton, and, of course, St. Thomas, a small town in Ontario, where he spent 12 long, character-building years.

There's not a week that goes by when someone at my hospital doesn't tell me of their appreciation for Thom's writing and his perspectives. He has written hundreds of columns for our local paper, *The Hamilton Spectator*. And I think one of Thom's strengths is seeing the wonder of today—seeing the tiger lilies on our neighbour's lawn and taking a moment to appreciate both the garden and the gardener.

Happy Birthday, Thom!

And, if you wish to enjoy Thom's columns from the Hamilton Spectator, visit or subscribe at www.thomasfroese.com.

Dear Friends: I pray that each day, birthday or not, you and I will each have new eyes to see the wonder of life and give thanks to the One who gives us the privilege to enjoy it.

Dr. Jean

July 26, 2020

14. On the Other Side of the Knife

This week I was happy to wear a mask. It helped me to avoid questions, like "What happened to your face?" With a strong family history of facial skin cancers, I couldn't ignore the small lumps on my nose and decided I'd better get them off.

I got an appointment with a very pleasant dermatologist here in Hamilton. I knew what was coming. You can't make a diagnosis without a biopsy. Of course, that meant a needle in the nose: slightly more painful than the COVID-19 swab testing, which many of us have recently experienced. The empathetic nurse who did the injection, was kind enough to tap the end of my nose as she was injecting. There's nothing like a little distraction to help one deal with searing pain.

On a more positive note, it is always good to be on the other side of what we health care professionals do to others, and my work certainly involves a fair number of diagnostic biopsies. Being on the opposite end of a blade helps ensure that I remain an empathetic doc.

All that to say, I was glad to wear a mask for the rest of the week and avoid awkward questions from my patients about the chisels on my face. In addition, I think having a haircut by an actual hairdresser also helped to improve my looks this week.

At the end of the long work week, Thom and I had a short anniversary getaway for the weekend, and we visited some of the significant landmarks that related to our wedding a short 19 years ago. That walk down memory lane included a visit to St. Thomas, Ontario, a once thriving railroad town. At the Elgin Country Railway Museum, we saw photos of the rail industry from 125 years ago.

Locomotive 999 boasted a speed that topped out a hundred miles an hour[11]. There was no question in everyone's mind at that time that she would remain as the leader in transportation for generations to come. Of course, no one knew that just around the corner, the automobile and then the airplane would leave her far behind on her own tracks in many parts of the world. Now in St. Thomas, one of the former busiest railroad lines ends at the museum, and there is no longer a functioning train station.

Our Long Midnight

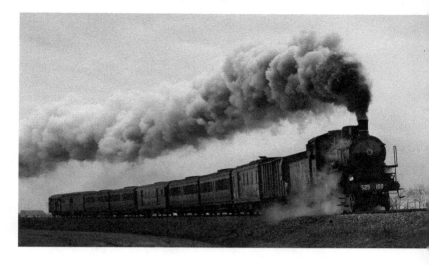

Adobe Images

The museum also had old photos of people: their stories and faces told the tale of their arduous lives and times. What made them struggle on?

It makes me wonder how the museums of the future will look at us today. With rockets that take us to the moon, how can we explain our global inequity? The photo below of this little Yemeni girl, who was a child bride in rural Yemen, tells quite a story about global inequity.

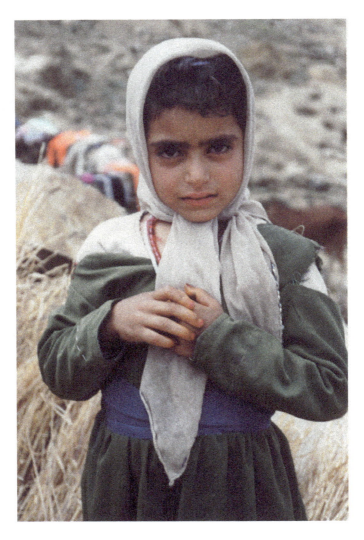

A child bride I met in rural Yemen (2006).

When I think about the current and past struggles of inequality and injustice, the centre line for me is the assurance that the Creator of each human life has a purpose and love for each one, whether in the past, present, or future.

Many would disagree with that concept, but for millions who have suffered over their lifetime, that confidence has given them dignity and hope. Random chance offers no comfort to grieving humanity. No matter who we are or where we live, each of us can raise our eyes and give thanks to our Creator. I believe that He became one of us in the person of Jesus Christ—whose personal story was full of mistreatment and even a brutal death. And now, as the Great Physician himself, who is stronger than death, He waits for us to invite Him to skilfully remove the lumps and bumps that each of us bear.

Dear Friends: You'll never regret the hands and work of the Great Physician. He gives us both healing and peace (Isaiah 53:5). That's a timeless gift for anyone.

Dr. Jean

August 10, 2020

15. Take the Plunge!

Well, he didn't exactly make a cannonball entrance, but after at least 10 years of not swimming, dad jumped into our pool and successfully reached the other end—doggy paddling all the way. He did look a little panicked by the time he put his hand on the other end of the pool, but he had a great smile of satisfaction. Mom has always been the swimmer in our family and with dad's more recent dementia, walking and other simple physical activities have been the cornerstone of his exercise routine. They do say that exercise is an important part of maintaining one's memory—so keep in good shape: a note for all of us.

Being cooped up in their little apartment / room for over 14 weeks has been challenging for them and other seniors. But on Friday, he did it! After a decade of not swimming, dad took the plunge at nearly 83 years of age and met the aquatic challenge.

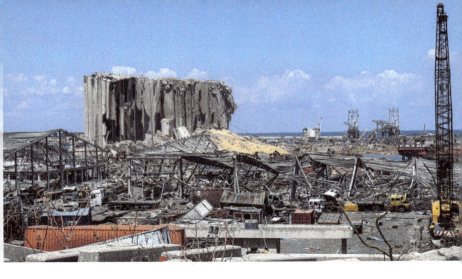

In Lebanon, more than 218 people were killed and 7,000 injured when 2,750 tons of ammonium nitrate exploded in Beirut's port on 4 August 2020.
Adobe images

I think of the many others who faced greater challenges this week—our dear global friends in Beirut, Lebanon who went to work one morning, only to have much of old city blow up in front of them. The first responders arrived with an ambulance: Who would they take first? Health workers, overwhelmed in the hospitals, were trying to triage and save as many lives as possible. They were thrown into chaos and forced to take the plunge, their strongest preparation being the smaller moments of challenge and strain that they had experienced as frontline workers. Emergency drills and protocols are helpful but could never have prepared them for something like this.

It makes me reflect on the openings we missed to stretch ourselves this week: to do the things that we knew we should do. Yet, we found it easier to sit on the side of the pool and watch someone else swim. Our stretch may be reaching out to a neighbour that we have never spoken to; applying for a work opportunity (whether paid or volunteer); asking for or giving forgiveness; or simply learning a new skill that will enrich our lives and that of others. The list goes on. We each can embrace one such chance and make the next step to taking the plunge, recognizing that the outcome isn't always predictable or easy. But the swim is worth it.

I am always encouraged that I don't ever swim alone. I can always call out to the Lord, who knows my strengths and weaknesses. He knows how far I can swim and exactly when he needs to reach down and lift me out of the water. If I was on my own, I would fear the outcome. But he reminds us that he knows the beginning and the end of everything, including the details of each of our lives. I am encouraged by the verse in Isaiah 41:10:

> So do not fear, for I am with you; do not be dismayed, for I am your God. I will strengthen you and help you; I will uphold you with my righteous right hand.

Dear Friends: I hope that you will take the plunge this week—whatever that looks like for you. Take a moment to write it down. Be encouraged by my 82-year-old dad, who left the safe edge of the pool and made it to the other side. You don't have to face the challenge alone. Our Father in heaven, through the hands of His Son Jesus, is reaching out to any of us who asks for His help.

Dr. Jean

September 1, 2020

16. Sow, Tend, Reap

I was pretty tired yesterday by the time I left the hospital at noon. I had worked all the previous night. But I was glad that, as I often do, I stopped on my way home to visit my folks in their seniors' residence. Often, we will go for a drive, and I called on capable driver Liz, my older daughter and an enthusiastic new driver, to help me out yesterday. Like many seniors, mom and dad just love to take a drive in the country.

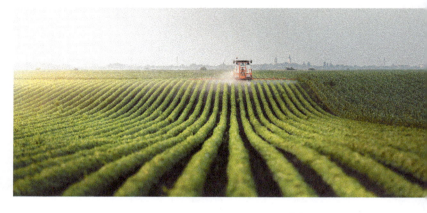

Adobe Images

Dad's background is agriculture and farming. On our frequent car rides in the country, we'll often drive close to the farmers' fields near Dundas, where we live, and simply observe the crops. Many years ago, I took these similar country drives with dad and his then 80-plus-year-old mother, who lived near London, Ontario. We'd often go crop gazing with grandma through the fields of Elgin County. Dad's reflections today about how good (or bad!) the crops look sound a lot like grandma's comments some forty years ago. All this crop gazing is giving me a profound appreciation for the patience of the farmer.

It makes me wish I had a little more of the farmers' patience: that confidence to plant choice seeds in the hard-tilled ground; the diligence to water and weed; and the discipline to effectively reap the crop and prepare it for sale. It all looks so easy as one races by the tall cornfields at a 100 kilometres per hour. But then we're simply observing the product and not appreciating the back-breaking steps that it took to get it.

Regardless of our location, I can't help but think that for many of us, this season of COVID-19 and of global strain is a lesson in agriculture. A simple lesson in sowing, tending, and reaping. Can we believe that at the end we will gain something valuable by planting at this difficult time? Can we keep watering the fields of our lives with life-giving water and intentionally applying the natural fertilizer and weed protection that will ensure a healthy product?

I bumped into a friend today in the hospital who was visiting her very ill father. Her dad had lived a life of impact and love, but now was struggling with significant disability and dementia. We briefly shared our stories of how difficult it was to see our fathers suffer. She wondered aloud if her visit to him made a difference. I reminded her of what she already knew: her caring for a vulnerable person always made a difference. She was sowing not only into his life but also into her own and into those who saw her commitment and love for an aging and disabled dad. She had an opportunity to make a difference that was not available for so many whose loved ones suffered from COVID-19.

Sow, tend, and reap.

It means intentionally ensuring that we invest in family and community, and actively weed out a spirit of entitlement or bitterness. It requires us to leave behind the comparing of ourselves with others and the excluding of those who are not like us. For me, cultivating these habits requires a new kind of person inside of me: a new perspective, one that I can't generate on my own. In his brief life on Earth, Jesus Christ lived this pattern perfectly. He sowed kindness and love. He tended to the vulnerable yet stood up boldly to his society's oppressors. In the end, because He suffered beyond imagination, He reaped the ability to give new life to anyone who asks Him for it.

Dear Friends: During this long season of COVID-19, may you know the fulfillment of sowing well in life and reaping the benefits that it brings.

Dr. Jean

September 13, 2020

17. Running with Purpose

I think many of us wake up some mornings and wonder what we are really doing here. Wonder what is the purpose of our individual or corporate lives? Do we just clock in our time and then check out at the appropriate moment, or are do we recognize that we here for a greater purpose that extends beyond ourselves?

I think of an elderly woman I saw in my medical office, who had a Niagara Falls' worth of tears running down her cheeks as she shared the hopelessness she feels due to her COVID-19 restricted life. She felt she had no purpose in her life; she could not enjoy her usual activities, and she feels utterly alone. I see more mothers coming in to deliver, who had no prenatal care, who are relying on addictive drugs to soothe their social isolation and fears during their pregnancy. It's a risky proposition for both them and their babies.

How does our purpose become restored? We can look to people like young Anne Frank[8] who, during the Second World War occupation of her city of Amsterdam, wrote captivating journals about hiding from the Nazis. These writings later become archives of history and a testimony of the endurance of a young Jewish teen and her family during dark times. Anne died in a concentration camp before they were ever published.

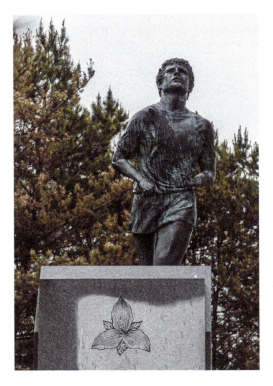

A monument of Terry Fox, a Canadian hero who changed the nation with his courage.
Adobe Images

Or we can look to Terry Fox, who became a Canadian hero.[9] While suffering bone cancer at age 17, and, after losing one leg, he began his long run across Canada to raise funds for cancer. The annual Canadian run in his memory is just around the corner, September 20. Forty years ago, his own cross-Canada run was cut short by a recurrence of his cancer, which quickly then robbed him of life at age 22. There were no more personal runs for Terry.

These are "legendary" examples of people who suffered in very difficult circumstances but somehow still remained centred in the meaning and purpose of their lives. Ironically, we are never promised to see the outcome of our life's purpose. Anne never imagined that her writings would be read by hundreds, let alone millions, and Terry did not know his runs have raised more than $800 million for cancer research. He hoped to raise just over $24 million.

Heroes often live in our community, our own circle. My father, who lost his own dad when he was only 16, beat the odds and went to university despite coming from a farming homestead where higher education was considered a waste of time. He walked through the challenges of raising a young family while pursuing further education. His latest season of life is tested by dementia and a failing memory.

During a video tribute to him and mom for their 60th anniversary this past Saturday dad's eyes welled up as he listened to many speak of the impact of his life on theirs. Dad was reminded of his life's meaning and purpose. He doesn't like what is happening to him now, but it doesn't diminish the impact he has made.

I was once asked during a TV interview[g] about my "centre line," that is what kept my own life in balance and filled with purpose, especially in my work abroad. My centre line is that I am created and loved by God. This gives me hope to move into difficult circumstances and really uncomfortable moments. And when I reflect on God's love for every other human being that I meet—regardless of their culture, beliefs, or background, I can see them as equally loved, created with a purpose.

Dear Friends: People and institutions will disappoint you. But your purpose in life will be centred when you know and embrace how much you are loved by the God of the universe. I hope that each of you will find that purpose in life and be able to live it out, even when the circumstances of life are shouting out against you. I personally find strength in the promise from Jeremiah 29:11 (NIV): *"For I know the thoughts and plans that I think toward you, says the Lord, thoughts of peace, and not of evil, to give you an expected end. Then you will call upon me, and you will go and pray unto me, and I will listen unto you."*

Dr. Jean

---

[g] "Made in Canada" (2012). Produced by Karen Pascal with Crossroads Communication: https://www.youtube.com/watch?v=4yLzt054A2g

September 28, 2020

18. Go Ahead and Flush!

If you live in a part of the country where the weather was pleasant for just one more week of the autumn season, then I hope you've enjoyed the persistent warmth. In addition, I trust you saw some of the trees that are already changing colours as we head toward the wintery snow and ice. Some of my friends who live in warm climates all year round may not understand how each little degree Celsius (and for our American friends, Fahrenheit) is so precious to us.

As I walked in the leaves with a friend this week, I was not reflecting on the colours, but on the need for each of us sometime in life to, well ... flush. Now when you are a gynaecologist, you probably have fewer inhibitions in talking about topics that are otherwise socially awkward. Flushing is one of those topics. We flush what we don't want to see again. We want what is flushed out of our sight and mind. I've never known of anyone who has (successfully) chased after what they've flushed.

Sometimes harmful words or negative experiences have played out in our lives. We have dealt with them with the appropriate response or action, but then, they are still just there. They can taunt us, haunt us, and make us sad or angry again. We recognize that we no longer want them to consume our thoughts and attention. The truth is, they simply need to be flushed.

We don't want to be like the cow, whose unchewed food goes to her first two stomachs and is stored there until she coughs up it (the 'cud') up and then chews it completely before swallowing it again. You get the point. The cow recycles and rechews her food, and it requires a lot of energy.

Is there something that you need to flush? I'm not talking about ignoring a wrong and sweeping it under the carpet. But if you've dealt with hurtful words or actions, you don't have to let them consume any more of your mental, spiritual, or emotional energy.

We each can experience the power of the flush: It's the power to rid ourselves of ruminating so an injustice can no longer consume our space. But we can also be freed from ruminating on our shortcomings and omissions, the times when we didn't choose the right way. Jesus Christ promises to remove them permanently from of our sight and reach. In addition, He gives us the strength to approach those whom we have wronged and try to make things right with them.

Circling back to the flush—I hadn't given much thought to the power of the toilet until a couple of my university colleagues introduced me more fully to the impact of not having a toilet. Drs. Corinne Schuster Wallace, Susan Watt, and Susan Elliott shed more light for me on what was happening around me as I lived and worked in East Africa. Have a look at the video that was presented to the UN headquarters in New York for World Toilet Day a few years ago.[h] (Yes, there is a World Toilet Day that is observed in November each year).

Dear Friends: As you enter the remainder of this week, I hope that you will flush at least once. Flush down what you don't need to chew on any longer. And be reminded of the great love and power of Christ to do the same for each of your shortcomings and failures.

Dr. Jean

---

[h] "Toilets and Safe Motherhood," a video presented by the United Nations University at the United Nations on World Toilet Day, November 19, 2014: https://www.youtube.com/watch?v=wZqbVebBCEI

October 12, 2020

19. The Power of Giving Thanks

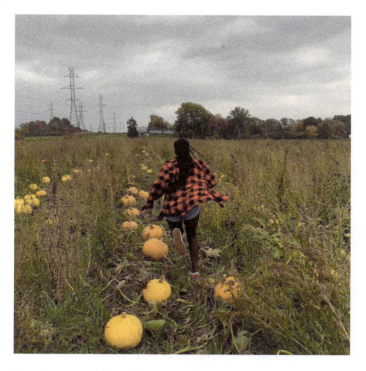

Daughter Hannah loved her visit to the pumpkin patch.
A safe outing during the pandemic.

We have had a unique Canadian Thanksgiving weekend. Canadians celebrate their Thanksgiving earlier than our American neighbours to the south. Unlike some of our American friends, we want to have our turkey before the snow flies.

I've spent many Thanksgivings at home and abroad waiting earnestly for the chance to meet with family around a turkey dinner. But this year, my older sister had to make the ominous COVID-19 announcement: Stay at home. No family gathering this weekend for the Chamberlain clan.

One thing I love about my husband, Thom, is his ability to make lemonade out of lemons. After my long Thanksgiving weekend day on call, instead of turkey, he offered to treat me to a really romantic evening with a 1950s movie *On the Waterfront*. It's a story about the power of the mob along the docks of New Jersey, with background big band music that was loud enough to beat back my fatigue.

My mom always loved these kinds of movies: a handsome guy with just a bit too much makeup and a love story with over-the-top drama. But if one can look past the 1950's nature of the movie, the theme of power, who has it and why, has some application to today. The powerful were the mob to be sure: People died at their hands while others who joined the mob, rose to incredible success at great speed. Power also brought down the untouchable mob, the power of consistent love and desire for change wielded by just a few. Dockworker Terry Malloy, along with his Catholic friend Father Barry, stood together and toppled the mob. They united Terry's fellow workers: Men who were consistently abused and living in fear. Terry was a "small" man who discovered a lot of power.

This makes me think of the power of Thanksgiving. It's a time that mysteriously brings together families and friends. Together we celebrate each other and the blessings of the year. Happy families, saddened families, rich and poor families— each gathering. We don't gather to celebrate our rights, our successes, or our entitlements.

Thanksgiving has its own mysterious power to bring people together and give us a new perspective on our circumstances.

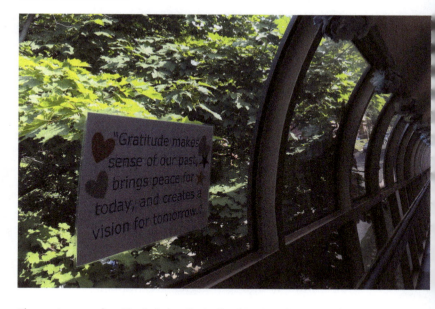

The posters on of gratitude lining the halls of St Joseph's Hospital, Hamilton, reminded staff, patients, and visitors of the power of Thanksgiving.

In contrast, I'm reminded of a fellow that I met while crossing the "bridge" that links the parking lot and the main part of St. Joseph's Hospital, Hamilton. In the early days of the COVID-19 crisis, kind volunteers had placed some positive messages in the windows of the bridge, along with blue puffy balls to bring a bit of colour to the sterile environment of the hospital. I greeted the man and commented positively on the new decor as we crossed the bridge. He mumbled with distaste that the balls remind him of the coronavirus. That certainly took the wind out of our conversation. We were looking at the same thing but with very different perspectives.

Some of our movies tell stories of people who, in very difficult circumstances or places, were able to harness the power of a thankful heart, and produce a positive change that benefited many. *Life is Beautiful* (1998), *The Hiding Place* (1975), *Gandhi* (1982) and *Schindler's List* (1993) are just a few.

Thanksgiving brings us together as families, as communities, as friends. We may not have gathered in large groups this weekend, but within our small "bubbles," that mutual expression of thanksgiving for what we have is a powerful perspective changer.

I'm grateful that we can also express our thanksgiving to the giver of life—the God of the universe who cares for each of His creations. He's the one who sees Hannah as she runs through the Thanksgiving pumpkin patch—filled with the energy of youth and a heart filled with thanks.

Dear Friends: How can you flex your power of Thanksgiving this week? Regardless of our circumstances or geography, we'll enjoy a healthier and more hopeful perspective if, each day, we celebrate one moment of thanks.

Dr. Jean

October 26, 2020

20. Commitment During Calamity

I didn't even know where to look for them. I hadn't put on my high heeled shoes in over half a year. There hasn't been an occasion to do so. No one can see my shoes on Zoom. But this past Saturday, my young nurse cousin was tying the knot with a handsome engineer, and Thom and I were invited to the wedding. I had texted her a few days before to ensure it was still an 'in-person' event. She assured me that with a church capacity of nearly 1000, they weren't going to be breaking any public health by-laws.

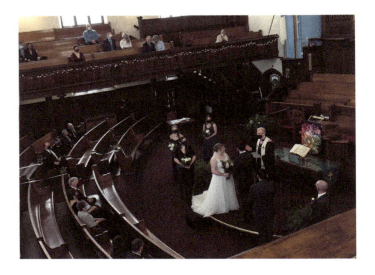

Guests spread out during the wedding ceremony of Heather Kell Rose and Tyler Fish at Ryerson Church in Hamilton, October 2020.

The beautiful morning arrived, and we all approached Ryerson Church in Hamilton, with smiles behind our masks and virtual hugs for beloved relatives who have been out of our "bubble" for what seems like a decade. We've all aged a bit. Some folks were absent due to illness, but as many as could responsibly gathered in the century-old church, to be part of this special day. We were scattered and spaced throughout the auditorium: many on the ground floor with the rest of us in the large encircling balcony. From there, Thom and I really had the real bird's-eye view. The ceremony was lovely, the vows were taken, the rings were given, and the papers were signed.

Everyone strolled out, though spaced apart, through the single front entrance to wish the groom and bride a happy life together, from a distance. Little wedding favours were packaged for each of us, which included a small container of chocolate milk (the bride grew up on a dairy farm) and an apple and cookie to sweeten our day.

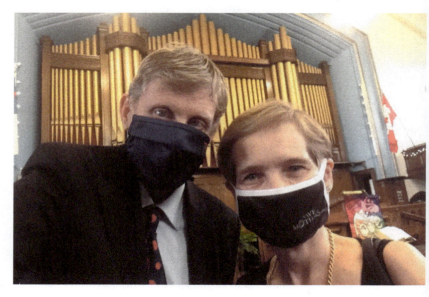

My husband Thomas Froese and I attend the wedding of my cousin Heather during the pandemic.

Thom and I drove off after taking our photos and, no surprise to those who know me well, I wanted to get out of my fancy shoes as quickly as possible!

On the drive home, we were reflecting on getting married during a pandemic—a COVID classic, one might call it. It was a wedding that was definitely challenging to arrange and may not have been all that the couple had ever dreamed. But in the hurdles and awkwardness of it all, this couple's simple commitment to one another was strikingly beautiful. They were promising their lives to one another, regardless of the circumstances around them.

I've heard of others who have done the same during these difficult times. They abandoned their lifelong dreams of a Cinderella wedding to simply commit themselves to a lifetime through the good and bad. A pandemic wasn't going to hold back their expression of love.

This reminds me of the commitment that our heavenly Father has made to us. He doesn't require all the pageantry and bells. He simply invites us to join Him in a life of love—to come, just as we are. To say to Him, yes, I will love you for my lifetime. He has already shown us His love through the unusual but selfless suffering of His Son Jesus. It seems like a paradox: Christ's suffering bringing our healing. I hope you have experienced that love and commitment during these challenging days.

So, congrats Heather and Tyler. We admire your love and promise to each other so beautifully seen by all of us who had the privilege to be there.

Dear Friends: My hope is that you have experienced another kind of love and commitment during these challenging days, the commitment that our Heavenly Father has for us. He doesn't require all the pageantry and bells. He simply invites us to join Him in a life of love to come, just as we are, to say to Him, yes, I will love You for my lifetime.

Dr. Jean

November 2, 2020

21. The New Look in Healthcare

It was Dress-up Day this past Friday at my hospital clinic. In the spirit of having some fun and boosting morale, I joined the very well-dressed office staff where I have the pleasure to work. The winner was definitely our office administrator, who hilariously suited up as an inflatable baby. I'll never see her the same way.

I dressed as a physician basketball player (a.k.a. myself) and my very competent and friendly nurse in a tutu. It's sure handy to have teenage kids whose outfits are easy to borrow and already coordinated. Costume contests have never been my forte. One new patient really did take a second look at us and wondered why the unusual outfits. I guess the world has been so turned upside down for her that she forgot it was Halloween weekend!

Dr. Jean Chamberlain-Froese

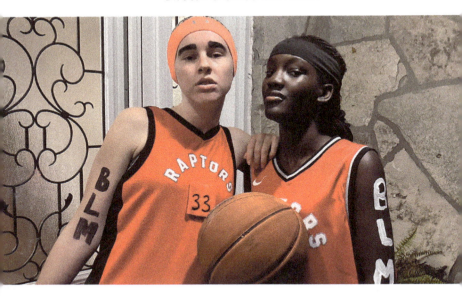

Liz and Hannah dressed for Halloween as basketball stars.

Yesterday (November 1st) was All Saints Day—the day that follows Halloween in some parts of the world. In some Christian traditions, it's an opportunity to give thanks for those who have gone before us in the faith, a time to celebrate that generational history.

In these times of global chaos, I think about the people—some of the saints—who have gone before us. I wonder how they would respond to such a crisis. I reflect on some of the nearly impossible things that they accomplished, the institutions they developed, and the sound principles they infused into our everyday lives. Even when we don't recognize them. Their resources were sparse, their technologies often simple, and their day-to-day life was difficult.

History often tells us about their mistakes—and there were many of them. They were not saints because of what they did, but rather who they were. They were children of God: simple people who had given up trying to win God's favour and instead had received His favour through the death and resurrection of God's son Jesus Christ. That changed everything for them. Their purpose in life, or raison d'être, became less entangled in their self-survival and instead was centred on bringing hope and healing in the darkest corners of the world. That journey took some to their own neighbourhood or village and others to places on the other side of the globe.

As I reflect on the saints who have lived before us, I am grateful that because of their example and words, each of us can also join in a fulfilling life as a saint. It's available for the asking—but hold on for the ride of your life!

Dear Friends: In this season of remembrance, we are thankful for those who have gone before us and reflect on what we are leaving behind.

Dr. Jean

November 15, 2020

22. It's Heating Up Around Here

I wish I could say that the temperature is going up in my Canadian province of Ontario. But the reality is that we're moving into winter, and the red that is coming is NOT warmth: it's the red zone of COVID-19.

Many countries are facing a similar challenge. Some also use colour-coded categories to describe their current viral status. For example, each region of Ontario, Canada is designated with a certain colour code or category: "The five categories are Prevent: (Green), Protect: (Yellow), Restrict: (Orange), Control: (Red), and Lockdown: (Grey)."[10]

As of today, my hometown of Hamilton has been designated as Red. It means more closures and restrictions, with gatherings being confined to 10 people indoors and 25 people outdoors.

The Red designation started in our neighbouring city Toronto, which is about 80 kilometres away along the coast of Lake Ontario, and has edged its way toward us here in

Hamilton. High numbers of COVID-19 cases abound—the count goes up with every daily newscast. It can be downright depressing.

It's interesting to see different people's responses to the change in colour coding (e.g., Orange transforming into Red). My daughter Liz would be happy to see all schools going virtual, while my daughter Hannah is almost in tears, hoping that schools will stay open and in-person. But it's not only the question of in-person or on-line schools.

The impact of this virus blindsided the young family of Gillian McIntosh.[11] She is a 37-year-old Canadian mother in an Intensive Care Unit (ICU) in Abbotsford, British Columbia, (in Western Canada). She was just delivered the other day by C-Section due to severe consequences of the COVID-19 virus. We're told by that even now, comatose in the ICU, Gillian doesn't even know that she has delivered her son. The baby has yet to be named. Her husband David holds their two-year-old Emma in his arms as he waits for his wife and baby son to come home. Gillian contracted the disease outside of hospital and was later admitted to the ICU with severe respiratory symptoms.

Thankfully, most mothers with COVID-19 and their babies do very well. But there are the unfortunate exceptions, like Gillian. These are difficult days and the path ahead for many around the world is uncertain. Our prayers are with Gillian and her young family.

Our Long Midnight

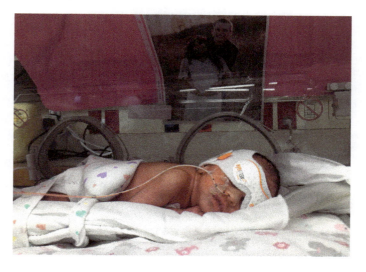

Premmie Hosanna Froese (no relation to Dr. Jean) who was born at 32 weeks when her mother, Preeti Froese, was ill with COVID-19. The baby spent 10 days in the NICU before her mom was able to visit her in person. During that time, Dr. Jean sent photos and video to Hosanna's parents, Preeti and Ben, (friends of Jean's through her church).
Used with permission.

Each of us has a unique story during this 21st century global pandemic. For the majority it includes many windows of uncertainty and even fear, both for the present and the future. Buckets of tears are shed, with few family or social gatherings to counter the balance. But during this time that feels like a worldwide wasteland, I hope that you will be able to lean into the promise that Jesus Christ offers to each one of us, regardless of our geography, gender, or age. It's not a promise to take away our problems and challenges, but rather that He will walk with us during this short course of life. There is much more yet to come. In the meantime, our heart and hands are secured when our little fists are clasped in His big hands.

I have many times held onto His promise: *"When you pass through the waters, I (God) will be with you; and when you pass through the rivers, they will not sweep over you. When you walk through the fire, you will not be burned; the flames will not set you ablaze"* (Isaiah 43:2).

Dear Friends: In the red and heat of your life right now, may you feel that strong hand around yours.

Dr. Jean

November 30, 2020

23. How Can You Be Mad at This Face?

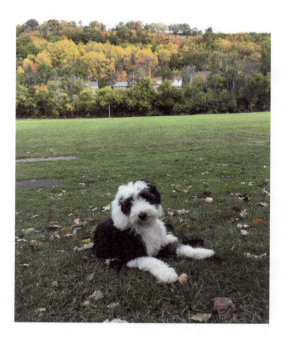

"Gracie Froese" relaxing in Dundas Park, Ontario.

I'm sure that you would never believe that this sweet little dog could ever torment an innocent person. Well, think again!

Just last week, our seven-month-old sheepadoodle had me on my knees, begging for mercy. Here's what happened. I had arrived home from the hospital late one evening and thought, "Why not stretch my legs after a long day and take the dog around the block?" I had a few little "treaties" in my hand: Never hurts to have a few in case the dog gets out of hand.

Well, that night she was "out of hand" as we walked. Not sure if one of the kids had gotten Gracie excited before I arrived home, but she wanted to push mommy's buttons. With one leap into the air and a sudden jerking on the chain, she was freed from my leash control. I immediately knew I was in trouble, and she was confident that her fun with mom was just beginning. Gracie started running circles around me. Any attempt to grab her collar was unsuccessful. Her long straight coat of hair hid her thin collar.

I tried to outsmart her with a bribe. Out came the treaties. No luck. Her circles started to get wider and included dangerous darts out onto the road. Cross Street was the name of the road. Fitting for how I was starting to feel. But I was also a bit nervous. Car lights were slowly turning at the street behind me. Thankfully, the driver could see what was going on: a desperate dog-owner was trying to get control of an out-of-control puppy. The driver stayed there beside us, motionless in his car, for a minute or two. Staring.

I eyed the nearby neighbour's home. Probably too far to go to try and get help. Of course, tonight I didn't bring my phone. Finally, I realized the only hope I had was to get moving. Crouching on the sidewalk with treats in my hand was getting me nowhere. I stood up straight and turned back toward home and shouted out a cheerful little call for the dog to follow. Finally! She took my bait. I heard the little paws behind my feet.

It was very dark. The streetlights flickered as we both trotted back to the house. I didn't dare look down. I could still hear the paws and kept running. I ran faster and faster, as if to challenge her to a race to get back home. I leaped onto the front porch, and she quickly followed. Eventually Thom brought out some cold-cut meats, dangling temptation at the end of his fingers.

Her mouth opened to take a bite and Thom had her. I almost cried! She was finally back in our arms and care. Thom placed her back in her little home within our home, on warm blankets.

As I recouped from my dog-trauma and near miss, I thought about human behaviours that might have parallels to Gracie's actions.

Her desire to be free from all restraints, to move in her own direction on her own time made me afraid and upset at the same time. After all, I was her guardian and protector. I just wanted her to come back to me. No questions. No hoops to jump.

Maybe I had a slight taste of how God feels when we step outside of His direction and limits. The tears are in His eyes because He knows we have such potential to harm ourselves. We want to fully explore our perceived rights and freedoms: there are so many options within our social circles, our sexuality, our relationships to mention a couple. As we widen our circle onto the road, He knows a car is coming around the corner. He calls, but we ignore Him. He begs, but we do not listen. He doesn't want to take away our fun or freedom, He just wants us back in His arms, safe and loved.

In *The Message*, Jesus expresses it this way:

> Come to me. Get away with me and you'll recover your life. I'll show you how to take a real rest. Walk with me and work with me; watch how I do it. Learn the unforced rhythms of grace. I won't lay anything heavy or ill-fitting on you. Keep company with me and you'll learn to live freely and lightly. (Matthew 11:28-30)

Dear Friends: Running around in circles makes us tired. In these dark times of our human experience, let us run into the arms that will never let us go. Being safe in the arms of God is not a limitation. It's a freedom to enjoy all that He has provided, giving us both strength and an anchor in our lives.

Dr. Jean

December 7, 2020

24. Lamenting the Holidays

Not many women look forward to visiting their gynaecologist— let's be honest. In a feeble attempt to divert the attention of anxious women, I usually make small talk with my patients. At this time of year, I commonly ask about their plans for the upcoming holiday season. But these days, I'm a bit reluctant to ask.

Not surprisingly, the discussion doesn't generate warm and cozy feelings of happy expectations. Rather for many, it is a reminder of sadness, loss, and loneliness. This is the world that we find ourselves in.

So far, over 280,000 people died in the United States[12]—our close neighbour to the south. That's over a quarter of a million people: These are the countable physical deaths in that country. But no one can accurately count the financial, emotional, and social deaths and the disabilities that have occurred in many countries ravished by COVID-19. Disappointment and loss are the holiday themes among many of our global citizens.

Looking at the situation in the world Jesus entered over 2000 years ago, the similarities with our loss of personal choices, freedom and livelihoods are astounding. The Hebrew people had lost their national autonomy and wealth, as had most countries in the region. The Romans ruled a large part of the known world, with their brutality and inhumanity. We may have hope in conquering the coronavirus (COVID-19), but to most of the world's population, the Roman empire seemed like an unstoppable brutal dictator. There was no hope for a vaccine next year to stop that global power. It would take much more than that.

A young single woman living in rural Palestine seemed completely incidental to the world issues at the time. She becomes pregnant—a social disgrace to her family and fiancé. In a moment, like a delicate china cup tossed carelessly on the floor, Mary's hopes for her future were dashed. The angel had had given her the promise of a new life and new hope by the angel. But at the moment, those words must have seemed very empty. In a dirty barn, far from her mother and family of origin, she experienced the pain of unaided childbirth. Not long after, the young couple and baby would flee as refugees, trying to avoid the King Herod's massacre of infant boys in Bethlehem.

Fast forward several thousand years: the Christmas story in the modern world has been made much more warm-hearted than the original. The bright lights, toys for the kids, and parties for all are often very attractive. But they don't evoke the despair and pain at the time of Christ's birth.

Our Long Midnight

I think this year is going to be different. People are sad, disappointed, and grieving.

But maybe it's the right time for many of us to look back to that miraculous moment. God becoming one of us, not as a person of privilege, but born in poverty, in captivity to a ruthless government, and in the middle of family disappointment.

That is the Christmas story, and it brings hope to our hopelessness when the lights, the gifts, the parties, and drinks simply cannot do it. God came to be one of us and to give His life to transform ours: to give us a life that will never end. Our sadness and disappointment are forever gone.

Because of this, our lives can be profoundly changed. Yes, we experience pain and at times, indescribable grief. But we don't have to bury that sadness or pretend it is not there. Instead, we are able to acknowledge that deep sadness and turn to the one who was called "a man of sorrows"—Jesus Christ. From a place of honour and comfort in heaven, He willingly took on pain, rejection, and isolation so that we could always look to Him who could honestly say, I know, I have been there.

Dear Friends: I love the lights of Christmas. They have never been more beautiful than this year. But as we see the lights shining in the darkness, my prayer is that you might look to the real light of Christmas, Jesus Christ, and know the life and peace that only He can give to each of us. Even in your sadness, look to His light.

Dr. Jean

December 14, 2020

25. Tired of Being Afraid?

I've performed surgery on many women during my nearly 25 years as an obstetrician/gynecologist. I don't remember many of them commenting on how happy they were to be operated on. Undergoing surgery and experiencing life altering change, like the loss of an organ, can generate a lot of fear, even if the change is for the better.

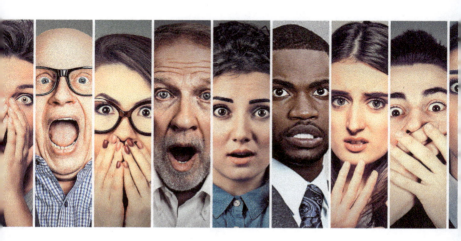

Adobe Images

Dr. Jean Chamberlain-Froese

Most of us have experienced fear in this year of 2020—the year that sounded so smooth and round in its enunciation and ease of writing. Twenty—Twenty. Maybe it would be better called Fear—Fear. Fear of contracting a fatal disease' fear of passing it on to vulnerable relatives' fear of political instability' and fear of social or financial collapse.

My sister-in-law had surgery this past week. She is convalescing at our home for a while. I'm engaged in nursing, personal support work, and trying to provide some palatable nutrition for her recovery. We talked about the surgery beforehand. She was understandably fearful. Would it work? Would it be painful? Would the surgeon carry out the right procedure (there was debate about the best approach for her failing knee)? Despite the fear, she took the steps and had the surgery.

After the procedure, she was in pain. And then came the fear of never getting better. The fear plays on our mind as we lay on our bed of recuperation. I'm sure many others recovering from COVID-19 right now also fear ongoing disability or disease. Some people may not have had the disease but fear for the future as they fear for today.

Fear is a powerful thing. It can incapacitate us. Fear of what will happen; fear of what HAS happened; and fear of the current shifting sand, or even of good things. Fear of starting a new relationship, finding a better or more suitable job, going back to school.

During the pandemic, our fears may also make us less likely to interact with others who are different from us.

On the news we hear and see the same perspective every day. Our fears are reinforced.

The story of Christmas, on the other hand, invites us into a world where we can set aside fear. A world where we can know true joy even in difficult times and see the whole world with its global needs and struggles.

An angel invited the poor shepherds to go and see the baby Jesus in a nearby barn. That angel, likely an imposing figure, began his invitation with the assurance: "Don't be afraid." He continued, "Because I bring you good news" (Luke 2:10).

After visiting the newborn, these shepherds were still poor, and still felt the cold of the Judean evening. They were still seen as inferior citizens and outcasts. But with their simple belief in the Saviour baby, they could put their fears in perspective. On that night, God had brought peace and goodwill for all people. And now, in our modern world, we are still seeing the unfolding of this story, the changes made evident by God's presence in our world. The story is far from over.

Often enough, we realize these changes through a sort of surgery in our spirits. Yes, at times, things need to be removed or replaced in our character or natural responses. But we don't need to fear. Jesus is the great physician, who brings healing and health to each one who comes to him.

That is not to say that we will all be healed completely in this life. Instead, that happens at the end of the story—in a place that he has promised to prepare for everyone who loves him. He said, in John 14:2: "I am going there to prepare a place for you. And if I go and prepare a place for you, I will come back and take you to be with me that you also may be where I am."

And there will be no fear. This is not just for a select small group, but for everyone who embraces His message. At Christmas and at any time, this is the promise of peace and goodwill toward all people.

Dear Friends: I pray that you will hear and believe the words of the angels: DO NOT BE AFRAID. It means not trusting your own capacity to manage your fear but rather to embrace the power of the life, death, and resurrection of that baby born on Christmas night many years ago. He is the great physician, who takes away our fear and the things holding us back.

As we look into the new year and leave behind 20–20, the year of fear-fear, my prayer is that we look forward to the One who brings hope and change in our lives, both now and forever.

Dr. Jean

January 3, 2021

26. One Last Look at 2020

When the big ball came down in Times Square in New York City on December 31, 2020, at 24:00:00, I didn't hear a lot of discussion about wanting more of 2020. The global consensus was: Glad that's done. Let's move on to new things and a more "normal" life'. But as I leave this year of chaos, sadness, and loneliness, I want to reflect on a mother whose story closed the end of this infamous year.

And yes, the babies continue to be born in the midst of uncertainty and difficulty. I was on call the other night and helped to deliver five little lives, but I didn't catch the New Year's baby—another colleague did. There's always a bit of fun competition amongst health workers as to which hospital delivers the first baby of the year.

Our first delivery in Hamilton made the local newspaper with an interesting comparison to the first baby born in Hamilton 75 years earlier (1946) on New Year's Day.[13] The man, Donald Loney, was born just months after the nuclear bombing of Hiroshima and Nagasaki, which contributed to ending the Second World War.

The Hamilton Spectator describes the newborn of 1946 as surveying or looking at the new atomic world. The sentiment of the average person at that time was similar ours: sadness, fatigue, and looking around the corner for hope.

Many around the world ended 2020 with the celebration of a young mother whose life and character has changed the world. The mother, of course, was young Mary—a teenager whose life would otherwise have not been celebrated like those of the billions of people who have lived before our generation.

As I was reminded recently by Tim Keller,[14] Mary was a thinker, questioning her divine pregnancy. God is not afraid of our questions, but still won't always fill us in. The angel didn't tell her that Joseph, her fiancé, would also be updated on the upcoming birth, or that foreign kings would come to worship and bring extravagant gifts for the boy. God gave her just enough information to know that He was with her.

And her response has resounded down through history: It is recorded in the first chapter of Luke, verse 38": "Let it be to me according to your word." In other words, Even without understanding everything, I'm willing to be part of God's bigger story or plan. Mary hadn't given a trite or ignorant answer.

Of course, the story of a single virgin girl who's convinced that an angel predicted that she would become pregnant, would be just as unbelievable then as it is now.

Mary also knew what was ahead: rejection by her friends and possibly family and most certainly being cut off by her fiancé, Joseph. But through her questioning, she had confidence that God is indeed God. Mary, even with fear and questions, was willing to be part of God's bigger story.

As we approach the new year, I wonder how willing we are to be open to the plans that God has for us. 2020 has been a year of disappointment, loss, and loneliness. Like you, this year has caused me at times to be turned upside down to the point of exasperation.

We wish each other a "Happy New Year" but there is no guarantee that it will be happy. But it can be one of hope and purpose. Even in the dark times, we are reminded that Christ has promised to be our light. His purposes for our lives are bigger than we will ever understand.

I'm sure Mary could never have imagined that people in 2021 would still know her name.

Dear Friends: As we wave goodbye to the never-to-be-forgotten year of 2020, I hope you will have the open heart and hands of Mary to embrace what God has planned for you in 2021, with the heart to say, "I am willing. May everything you said come true."

Dr. Jean

January 10, 2021

27. On Turning 15

So our "little" girl Hannah turns 15 today. I hesitate to use the word "little" as none of my family members are smaller than I – save the dog. I am assured she won't surpass 35 pounds and even on her back legs standing tall, will always remain shorter than I am.

Hannah turned 15 in this week, the week of the storming of the United States Capitol in Washington DC. It will not easily be forgotten and has shaken many of about the world's longest continuous democracy and what should be respected and revered despite our differences. My husband, Thom, always ensures that as a family we watch these global events on the TV—we all sit together and reflect--to help the kids learn from the present as they live into the future. Sometimes the lesson is hard to grasp.

I was not at Hannah's birth, mother as I am and obstetrician as my profession. Hannah joined our family as an orphaned girl at the age of four. We visited her birthplace Mbarara hospital, Uganda, several years later. We had waited a few years to ensure that she would be able to remember the visit. We spoke with midwives and health workers who, though over a decade had passed, were able to give her some glimmers of light and history around her birth.

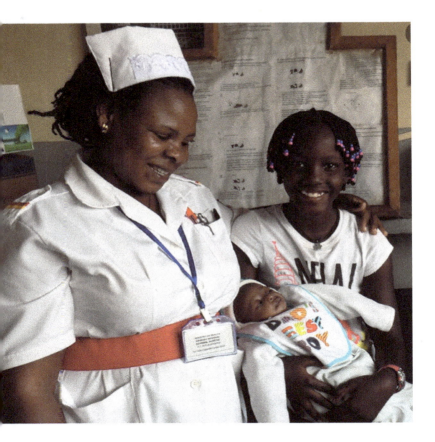

Hannah Froese meets Ugandan midwife Judith in 2017 at Mbarara hospital where Hannah was born in 2006.

Our Long Midnight

Midwife Judith told Hannah that her birth mom had arrived at the hospital in labour. She had been on a bus travelling through Mbarara with Rwanda as her probable destination. But she wouldn't make it that far. She was in labour and would deliver Hannah later that day. With limited supplies in the hospital and a need to identify whose baby was whose, most mothers would cut a small piece of their bed linen (usually a colourful sheet from their home) and tie it around the infant's small wrist. The mother's sheet matched the baby's bracelet. A simple solution when no identification bracelets were available. Hannah's birth mom did the same.

The next morning Hannah's birth mom quietly slipped away, knowing for her own reasons that she couldn't care for her infant. She was never to be seen again by hospital staff. But the midwives knew who the small baby was and they called her "Hannah." She was later transferred to an orphanage many hours away, where she lived for the early years of her life. The story of how Thom and I connected with her is another post to be written.

But today as I see this beautiful teen girl sing and dance during our family karaoke, I am reminded of who Hannah really is. She is not only our adopted daughter, but she is now a Ugandan-born Canadian and a young person who has experienced the many corners of the world, both geographically and economically.

But her real identity is that she is deeply loved by the God of the universe, who has a special plan for her life. The big picture of her life and purpose goes far beyond what we as parents and those close to her can ever imagine.

Hannah has embraced the never-ending life that Christ promises to each of us who receive it from Him freely. It's not a life earned or based on our being "good" but one to simply be received with thanks. I see the thankfulness that Hannah demonstrates as such a strong impetus in her living the kind of life that God has planned for her.

She's learning to use her voice—not with judgment or hate – but with clarity and justice for those who need it. Even tonight, her birthday movie of choice for the family was *Hairspray.* uses song and dance to help break down discrimination against people who are Black and those with larger body structures. Hannah keeps the message alive and meaningful even in her own home.

So, on this your happy 15th birthday Hannah, be reminded of whose you are. Your dad and I will always love and cherish you but your true identity is rooted in the love of the One who made you and has a special purpose for your life. In the meantime, we'll keep cheering you on.

Dear Friends: I know that few of us on Facebook are 15 years old (as my kids constantly remind me) but each of us can struggle with who we are, especially in times of change, loss, and grief. I pray that you will also be reminded of who you are. Christ invites each of us into the arms and safety of His Father.

Dr. Jean

January 18, 2021

28. When the Streets are Empty

This past weekend, I left a few minutes late to get to my shift at the hospital. Usually, I don't mind when the streets are empty and I'm trying to make up for lost time. Fewer cars and slow-moving pedestrians can sometimes take a couple of minutes off my journey. But this weekend, I felt different: I almost wanted to see more cars and dog walkers. Instead, I could only hear the eerie quiet of silent streets and feel the squeeze of a shrinking community.

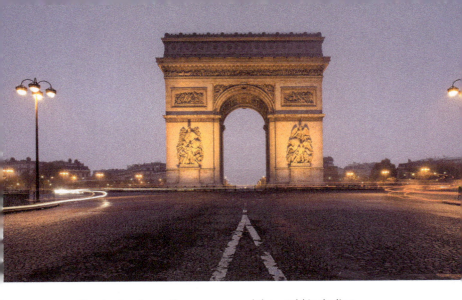

Empty streets are the norm around the world including usually busy tourist locations like the Arc De Triomphe in Paris.
Adobe Images

Everyone had been told to stay home, stay distanced, and not to go out unless necessary. It's all part of the second Ontario lockdown to reduce the increasing numbers of COVID-19 infections and deaths. The upward graph is starting to level out and we're all hoping to see a significant decline. Nonetheless, the Canadian evening news spends a lot of airtime discussing the COVID-19 pandemic from Eastern to Western Canada, with a brief update from around the world.

But as we know, COVID news is more than just statistics. My patient shared how her mother died recently of COVID-19 in the northeast USA. She didn't even get a chance to say goodbye to her. My role as a gynaecologist is sometimes to simply listen.

Her story made me a little more thankful for the opportunity that I have as an essential visitor to see my parents in their seniors' residence. Dressed up in "PPE" (who ever knew what "personal protective equipment" meant before March 2020?). Looking like an astronaut, I enter their room and provide some physical assistance and some simple communication with the outside world. Like many, my folks are frustrated that they can't leave the residence except for a short walk outside. We're counting the days until they get their vaccine and, in the meantime, keep following the guidelines to reduce the spread of COVID-19.

For now, their physical community is the people inside the residence, along with my sister Laura and me, who are their "essential visitors." Before COVID-19, we probably never gave much thought to anyone's virtual community. But for mom and dad, and many seniors like them, family and friends who send a text, telephone, or FaceTime, make up their essential connection with the "bigger" world. Mom and dad can't wait to see a video of great granddaughter Makinley—who is 120 kilometres away.

Flexible and diverse as a community may be, it is probably one of the most vulnerable assets we have during this global pandemic. In societies where people are more individualistic and less communal in their living, we have gained a much clearer awareness of the role of community in each of our lives. Fortunately, we've never had better communication tools for speaking to one another remotely. I remember the Saturday morning cartoon series "The Jetsons," which imagined that people could actually see one another on a TV screen. Well, we've surpassed that; the image is in our palms!

Despite these tools, many people are still very isolated during this global tragedy. It's hard to imagine why. I wonder if we become lethargic or just simply forget to connect with those who have a small or fragile circle of community around them. Electronic communication is rarely as effective as in-person but it's certainly better than nothing at all.

In addition, it is a quieter time for many to connect with our Creator. For some, it's hard to imagine that He is interested in us, if He even exists at all. But interestingly, the original story of this globe's history as described in the first book of the Bible, Genesis, tells of how God enjoyed walking daily and talking with the first two people He had made.

It might be a stretch to say God was lonely, His visits do reflect His love for community. Later in the Bible, He calls human beings "His friends"—people like Abraham, who simply believed who God was. That is where their friendship started. I hope you will take the moments to nurture a lifelong friendship with God.

Dear Friends: As we gaze into the fears and hopes of this next week, let's reflect on the importance of community, of being intentional about it and of including others who may struggle to be part of such a community. Who can you or I call today to remind them they're a valuable part of our world?

Dr. Jean

January 25, 2021

29. It's a Real Shame

She sat in my office this past week with tears welling up in her eyes. She felt shamed and blamed. My patient was pregnant and had unfortunately contracted COVID-19 early in December 2020. Positive patients usually have a special room, and appropriate PPE is used. The staff were not aware of her status so protocols had not been observed and numerous people wondered if they had been exposed. By the end of the visit and numerous calls to public health, it was sorted that my patient had not placed the clinic staff at risk of exposure. But for the first 45 minutes, tensions were high, especially as her husband had also attended (a "no-no" during the early COVID pandemic), further compounding the situation for possible exposures.

But here we were, at least six weeks later and the patient still felt traumatized. Through the tears, she cried, "I feel blamed for having COVID. As a PSW I was just doing my job at the nursing home and then I got sick." Of course, I spent the next several moments assuring her that no one blamed her for her positive COVID-19 test.

Our entire team was grateful for her work in a nearby seniors' residence. We only want what is best for her and her unborn baby. In my follow-up call with the patient and her husband the next day, I echoed the same message to him.

I reflected on my own experience of having a positive test myself before Christmas. I felt like an atomic bomb had gone off. Due to my recent heavy work schedule in the hospital, hundreds of people's Christmas and holiday plans were affected by my status. I was retested two days later due to uncertainty around the validity of the first test, only to find that I was not positive. But the knock-on effect of my status had caused several staff to be sent away from hospital duties early and my own parents were quarantined until only a few minutes before Christmas Eve dinner at their residence. It is easy to see how one can feel shame and isolation when tested positive for COVID-19.

This experience with my patient got me thinking a bit more about shame and its close, but distinctly different, first cousin, "guilt." Shame is a painful feeling that's a mix of regret, self-hate, and dishonour. "The same action may give rise to feelings of both shame and guilt; the former (shame) reflects how we feel about ourselves, and the latter (guilt) involves an awareness that our actions have injured someone else."[15]

From an awkward but practical point of view, shame can be used as an extremely powerful tool in modifying people's behaviour and providing social cohesion. It's been a sad but repetitive part of human history for a long time, including shaming by public floggings and shaving the heads of non-conformists. But invalid shame—arising from no action of the person themselves—has been heaped on millions of innocent people around our globe: shame for their ethnicity, their physical or mental challenges, their faith and gender. The list could go on.

Shame needs an antidote—a medicine to counteract its poison on individuals, who did nothing to invite this painful social disgrace. Some of us can play a part in helping to heal this toxin in other's lives by acknowledging their pain and preventing ongoing hurt. By promoting friendship and acceptance instead of rejection. It may even require us to examine how our treatment of others (whether intentional or not) can lead to feelings of shame.

I couldn't take away my patient's shame, but I could try to defuse its impact on her outlook and thinking.

In addition, I believe the antidote can be found through a relationship with the person who loves each of us for exactly who we are, Christ, because He personally knows the power and devastation of shame. He experienced unprovoked shame when He was unjustly condemned and inhumanely crucified.

His message is that He loves us regardless of how others have treated us and that he accepts us regardless of how we have treated others. Seems almost too good to be true, but He said it himself. Jesus used the example of a doctor to make his point that He is looking for those who have been shamed or rejected by the best of society: "People who are well do not need a doctor, but only those who are sick. I have not come to call respectable people, but outcasts" (Mark 2:17).

Dear Friends: I wonder if we could reflect for a moment on someone in your circle or community (including yourself) who has experienced invalid shame. My hope is that instead of self-hate and shame, they, or you, will experience the true acceptance and love that the great physician, Jesus Christ, offers to whoever will come to him.

Dr. Jean

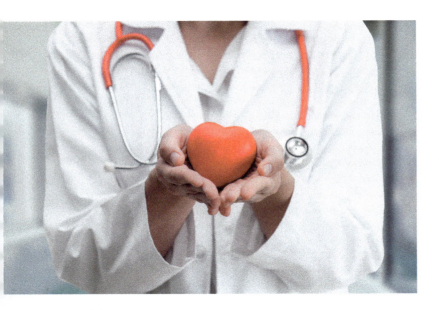

Adobe Images

February 1, 2021

30. Time, Love, and Tenderness

After seven years of slugging through an undergrad degree (biochemistry of all things!) and then earning my medical degree from the University of Toronto, I was ready for a real vacation. Before starting the challenges and long nights of internship, my graduating buddy, Dr. Bernadette Tran (otherwise known as "Bernie") and I decided in the middle of June, to drive to Florida for a holiday. I think the toils of medical school must have altered our judgment: driving in my parents' red Ford Mustang, with no air conditioning and only one of us licensed to drive the 24 hours in the 2200 kilometres of hot air and sun, was a decision I soon started to regret.

Bernie was wonderful moral support but couldn't help with any of the long drive in the 30 degrees Celsius (86 degrees Fahrenheit) weather. What did get me through (other than a lot of McDonald's coffee down Interstate 75), were the songs of the singer Michael Bolton. Bernie had all his songs on cassette tapes. Michael's beautiful voice kept me humming along with my eyes open. The one song that stuck out most vividly was "Time, Love, and Tenderness." It was the cure for a broken heart.

Yes, a lot of time has gone by since those days in the fiery red Mustang, but the need for time, love, and tenderness hasn't changed.

Time has been hard on most people during the pandemic: our faces are thinner with worry and drained by hospital masks. Some are heavier due to lack of exercise. My hands have aged and are constantly fighting the corrosive power of the ubiquitous hand sanitizer—thank you, Purell, and others, even if the constant sanitizing causes red itchy rashes.

Millions of us will have to heal from much more than a rash on their hands. It will take significant time to heal the many deep wounds. And healing doesn't mean without scars.

Some people especially feel the loss of time. For the young amongst us, the irreplaceable moments of graduations, birthdays, athletic awards, and simple times together with friends are the greatest losses. For others, seeing their loved ones for the last time or holding their grandchild in the first few days of life are paramount.

Our Long Midnight

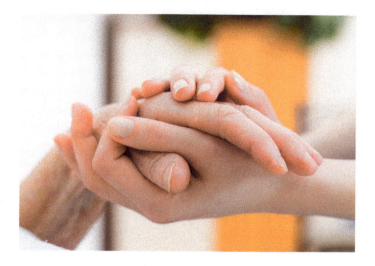

Adobe Images

We can never make up the time, but the healing is better when soaked in love and tenderness. I think of Mary Sardelis, who showered love on her 98-year-old mother, who lived in the long-term care home Park Place. Mary moved to care for her mom Voula, who was sick and dying with COVID-19. At the risk of her own life and facing the possibility that she may have failed, Mary demonstrated a purposeful and dedicated love for her mom. See the footnote below for her story.[i]

---

[i] CBC National, January 13, 2021. Story of Mary Sardelis: https://www.youtube.com/watch?v=kjYQDWjvyOs

Mary's example of selfless love has been repeated all over the globe, in many health care settings and beyond, even as we have been robbed of time. It's a reminder that time is a gift. It's never a certainty.

But as I reflect on time, I think of the one who holds all time in His hand, who called himself "the beginning and the end" (Revelation 22:13), that is Jesus Christ. Yet, as a human being himself, he experienced the realities and limitations of time. In the moments that he spent on this globe, he modelled perfect love to those who loved him and those who hated him. With tenderness, he forgave even those who even brutally killed him. He shared with us what it means to be human and offers each of us love and acceptance in a timeless eternity with Him.

Dear Friends: My prayer is that each of you will experience time, love, and tenderness this week—wherever your journey takes you.

Dr. Jean

February 14, 2021

31. Thank You Saint Valentinus for the Love

So, it's 20 years ago today that I said the big "Yes" to a young Thomas Froese, who requested my hand in marriage. It was quite an elaborate set up—our whole engagement—in London, Ontario.

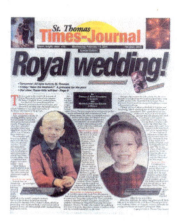

The front page of the St. Thomas Times-Journal (a mock copy) February 14, 2001, announces the wedding of Jean Chamberlain and Thomas Froese.

Not surprisingly, the story included 12 roses, a candlelit dinner for two, and a ring in the box. What was not so predictable was the 250-pound town crier who shouted out the big question in a restaurant filled with slightly irritated romantics and the radio announcement of our engagement only a few minutes after the question. And more surprisingly was the front page of the local newspaper in the hands of 50 or so actors at a nearby theatre proclaiming the marriage of the upcoming prince and princess, that is Thom and I. Thom spent a lot of energy in bringing this whole tale together, and it left many of his friends wondering how they could ever top his creativity and romanticism.

In hindsight, it was a good thing that he put all of his focus into this proposal, because the "Yes" response led to a 180-degree turn for him. We would be leaving our home and native country of Canada to live in Yemen, to learn not only how to live in a different culture and start a new job in a foreign language, but to also how to live a life as a newlywed couple.

This stretching experience helped us to learn to pull side-by-side in the same direction, even when we may have seen any given issue differently. I know that many of you have experienced this in your own relationships and marriages. For Thom and me, it was great practise for the rest of our married lives together to be reminded of the power of love in both the happy and sad times and the moments of victory and perceived defeat.

I guess we can thank Saint Valentine for his example. If you're familiar with the history, you will know that Saint

Valentine, rather known as 'Valentinus' was actually a Roman priest who was martyred by Emperor Gothicus around 269 AD. Saint Valentine's love[16] was for the person who had shown him the ultimate example of love: Jesus Christ. Jesus had loved those who others found unlovely, like the lepers that He healed. He cared and prayed for the needs of those who hated and hurt Him (even healing the cut ear of a man who came to arrest and kill Him).

It's true— the origins of Valentine's Day are not founded in a story of romantic love, but rather in selfless love, which can inspire all of us today. As the old song "What the World Needs Now" says, "What the world needs now is love, sweet love."[17]

In these days of struggle and international conflicts, avoidable and unavoidable human suffering and hunger, the need is true and selfless love. It means reaching out and helping those who cannot help us back.

I think of a Canadian couple named Steve and Peggy Foster who have spent their entire career in Angola, over 40 years. Steve is a talented surgeon and was one of the first graduates from McMaster Medical School. They raised their kids in Angola and are still there working today, showing compassion and care for anyone who walks through the door of their hospital. Even in times of war and danger, Steve and Peggy demonstrated unconditional care and love for both the victims and the perpetrators, even at the risk of their own safety.

When I think of Steve and Peggy, I see an example of Jesus Christ being played out in our present and difficult reality. Jesus said it plainly: "Your love for one another will prove to the world that you are my followers, my disciples" (John 13:35).

So Happy Valentine's to each of you and especially to my husband of 20 years—Thomas Froese. It's been an amazing journey.

Dear Friends: As we celebrate our love for those in our close circle, whether romantic, friendship, or family, may we also demonstrate selfless love that can do good for those who misunderstand or even hate us.

Dr. Jean

March 1, 2021

32. Riding the Wave

I don't need another wave in my life. I'm sure, like you, I'm not loving the idea of the "third wave" of COVID-19 that many experts predict. We've had enough ups and downs from the tidal wave of COVID-19. Another surge, and the fallout may seem more than many can bear.

I can hardly believe that it was one year ago today that I was flying back into Canada with a small team of friends and family, having just visited Uganda. We took no special precautions; it was just "business as usual" except for the occasional masked traveller in the international airports. At the time, the masks seemed like overkill in response to the mysterious viral infection that appeared confined to only a few areas of the world. But it would only be a few short weeks before we too would be donning the masks and restricting our own movements and activities.

I'm happy to report that in the Hamilton area where I live, we have now moved out of the "stay at home order" (sorry Toronto, Peel and North Bay/Parry Sound and other regions), so we are now able to meet in small groups. Faith communities can also meet if they enforce strict public health measures. At our local assembly, the young woman leading the music yesterday (Sunday) morning spoke about "surfing." What a perfect analogy it for our current situation. A surfer isn't drowned by the water if they stay on top of the powerful waves.

For a split second, the word made me think of the old TV series *Magnum P.I.*, about a private investigator who lived in Hawaii. Despite the rather cheesy story lines in nearly every episode, it had gorgeous scenery of Hawaii, and especially of the breathtaking waves with surfers making their way toward shore. These athletes had skill and power to stay on top of the wave and they had a durable board beneath them to bring them to safety.

I think we have all had a lot of practice in learning to be strong in difficult circumstances over the past year. It's been a very long work out. Recognizing that it is far from a perfect analogy, I wonder what the board is beneath us that keeps each of us afloat. For me, my feet are planted in the security and safety of Jesus Christ. He promises to be with us in the ups and downs of life, not only in this current pandemic but in the challenging moments of our futures. He was human and knew what it felt like to cry at the death of a friend and he also experienced the pain of torture and inhumane treatment at the hands of his enemies.

He only asks us to believe that he can give each of us a new start in life regardless of our past mistakes or present circumstances. It's profoundly simple but has changed the lives of people across this globe.

Dear Friends: We can ride the waves of this pandemic and the inevitable storms beyond it, with the assurance of Jesus' strong presence and footing in our lives. He not only understands the waves; He can even calm them.

Dr. Jean

References

1. The Holy Bible, New International Version. Grand Rapids: Zondervan Publishing House. 1984. Jeremiah 29:11 See www.biblegateway.com Quotes from the Holy Bible references in this book are taken primarily from the New International Version.

2. Jesus Calling Daily Devotional [Internet]. Sarah Young; c2020. Jesus Calling: [cited 2020 April 5]. Available from: https://www.jesuscallingdailydevotional.com/2019/08/jesus-calling-october-17th.html

3. Springer Rita, Fieldes Mia, Benjamin-Korporaal Bede. Midnight [song]. Light. Tennessee: Capitol CMG Publishing, 2020.

4. Tomlin Chris. Good Good Father [song]. The Ultimate Playlist. Tennessee: Capitol CMG Publishing, 2016.

5. Spafford Horatio, Bliss Philip. It Is Well With My Soul [song]. First published in Gospel Hymns No. 2. Chicago: Ira Sankey and Philip Bliss, 1876.

6. Crouch Andraé. The Blood Will Never Lose Its Power [lyrics]. Minnesota USA: Manna Music, 1966.

7. Henao Luis Andres, Merchant Nomaa, Lozano Juan, Gellder Adam [internet]. "A long look at the complicated life of George Floyd." 2020 June 11 [cited 2020 June 14]. *Chicagotribune.com*. Associated Press.

8. Wikipedia: the free encyclopedia [Internet]. St. Petersburg (FL): Wikimedia Foundation, Inc. Anne Frank. cited 2021 Jun 25. Available from: https://en.wikipedia.org/wiki/Anne_Frank

9. Wikipedia: the free encyclopedia [Internet]. St. Petersburg (FL): Wikimedia Foundation, Inc.; Terry Fox. [cited 2021 Jun 25]. Available from: https://en.wikipedia.org/wiki/Terry_Fox

10. Follert J. Ontario unveils new colour-coded COVID framework: Here's what that means for Durham Region. DurhamRegion.com [Internet] 2020 Nov 3 [cited 2021 Jul 8]. Available from: https://www.durhamregion.com/news-story/10238098-ontario-unveils-new-colour-coded-covid-framework-here-s-what-that-means-for-durham-region/

11. Nair R. B.C. mother who gave birth while in a coma due to COVID-19 is awake, meets baby for first time. CBC News [Internet]. 2020 Dec 16, [cited 2021 Jul 8] Available from: https://www.cbc.ca/news/canada/british-columbia/abbotsford-mcintosh-update-1.5844501

12. Institute for Health Metrics and Evaluation [Internet]. Seattle WA: University of Washington; c2020. COVID-19 Projections for United States of America; 2020, December 7th [cited 2021 Jul 8]. Available from: https://covid19.healthdata.org/united-states-of-america?view=cumulative-deaths&tab=trend

13. Van Dongen M. Hamilton's first New Year's baby is a symbol of hope — in any year Hamilton Spectator [Internet]. 2021 Jan 2 [cited 2021 Jun 25]. Available from: https://www.thespec.com/news/hamilton-region/2021/01/02/hamiltons-first-new-years-baby-is-a-symbol-of-hope-in-any-year.html

14. Gospel in Life. Mary's son: Timothy Keller [sermon on the Internet]. 2020 Dec 23 [cited 2021 Jul 10]. Available from: https://podcast.gospelinlife.com/e/marys-son/

15. Burgo J. The Difference Between Guilt and Shame. Psychology Today [Internet]. 2013 May 30 [cited 2021 January 25]. Available from: https://www.psychologytoday.com/ca/blog/shame/201305/the-difference-between-guilt-and-shame

16. Bitel L. The Real St Valentine was no patron of Love. The Conversation [Internet]. 2018 Feb 13 [cited 2021 Jul 25]. Available from: https://theconversation.com/the-real-st-valentine-was-no-patron-of-love-90518?gclid=CjwKCAiAsaOBBhA4EiwAo0_AnCo0xsPxIfOYrDRH0cHiX1pccWGp0KQMU_2sTULG0mJw7x1A4ZAhxBoCosQQAvD_BwE

17. David H, Bacharach B. What the World Needs Now Is Love [song]. New York: Blue Seas Music, 1965.

Additional Resources

Videos and songs from "Our Long Midnight"

a. "Jesus." 1979. The Film. Available at https://www.jesusfilm.org/watch/jesus Produced by John Heyman.

b. "Risen." 2016. The Film. available at https://www.youtube.com/watch?v=tgM1WGFTtjE directed by Kevin Reynolds.

c. Midnight. Song by Rita Springer https://www.youtube.com/watch?v=-9sbYnl3JrA From album "Light."

d. Video about having a baby during COVID (from St Joseph's Hospital, Hamilton, Ontario Canada. Produced by Dr. Jean Chamberlain) at https://www.stjoes.ca/health-services/women-s-infants- (click on 'Having your baby during COVID-19' video) or see https://www.youtube.com/watch?v=cduSDQdLTQM&t=4s

e. No Longer Slaves. 2018. Song by Zach Williams https://www.youtube.com/watch?v=bDnA_coA168 From album "Survivor."

f. Pandemic wolf stalks developing world. By Thomas Froese. (The Hamilton Spectator – Saturday, May 23, 2020) https://www.thomasfroese.com/pandemic-wolf-stalks-developing-world/

g. The Tyler Merritt Project. Before you call the cops. https://www.youtube.com/watch?v=oGu_xGBekpo or https://www.facebook.com/thetylermerrittproject

h. "Made in Canada" (2012) Produced by Karen Pascal with Crossroads Communication. https://www.youtube.com/watch?v=4yLzt054A2gw

i. Toilets and Safe Motherhood. Video presented by the United Nations University at the United Nations on World Toilet Day. November 19, 2014. https://www.youtube.com/watch?v=wZqbVebBCEI

j. Story of Mary Sardelis from CBC News. The National. January 13, 2021 https://www.youtube.com/watch?v=kjYQDWjvyOs

CPSIA information can be obtained
at www.ICGtesting.com
Printed in the USA
BVHW062256130222
628717BV00004B/27